This item must be returned on or before
the date stamped below.

Vignettes for the MRCOG

Edited by
Roy G Farquharson MD FRCOG

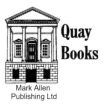

Quay
Books

Mark Allen
Publishing Ltd

Quay Books, Division of Mark Allen Publishing Group,
Jesses Farm, Snow Hill, Dinton
Nr Salisbury, Wiltshire, SP3 5HN

British Library Cataloguing-in-Publication Data
A catalogue record for this book is available from the British Library

ISBN 1-85642-056-6
© Mark Allen Publishing Limited 1998

Printed in the United Kingdom by Antony Rowe Ltd, Chippenham

618·0076
F

T04675

Contents

Contents

List of Contributors

Dr SA Walkinshaw is Consultant in Maternal-Fetal Medicine at the Fetal Centre in Liverpool Women's Hospital, L8 7SS

Dr RG Farquharson is Consultant Gynaecologist at Liverpool Women's Hospital, L8 7SS

Professor W Prendiville is Associate Professor in the RCSI Department of Obstetrics and Gynaecology at Coombe Hospital, Dublin, Eire

The late Professor MC White was Professor of Medicine at the University of Hull

Dr EI Turner, formerly Registrar in the Department of Clinical Biochemistry, Royal Infirmary, Edinburgh EH3 9YW, is now at the Killin Medical Practice, Laggan Leigheas, Perthshire FK21 8TQ

Dr ARM Sproston is Clinical Research Fellow in the Cancer Research Campaign Department of Experimental Radiation Oncology, Paterson Institute for Cancer Research, Christie Hospital, Manchester M20 9BX

Mr R Kingston is Consultant Gynaecological Surgeon and Oncologist in the Department of Gynaecology, Liverpool Women's Hospital, Liverpool L8 7SS

Dr Z Alfirevic is Senior Lecturer Consultant in Obstetrics and Gynaecology in the Department of Obstetrics and Gynaecology, Universiy of Liverpool

Mr H Gee is Senior Lecturer in the Department of Fetal Medicine, University of Birmingham

Dr K Sharif is Research Fellow in the Department of Obstetrics and Gynaecology, University of Birmingham

Dr SV Jones is Senior Registrar in the Reproductive Medicine Unit, Liverpool Women's Hospital, Liverpool L8 7SS

Dr RJ Armatage is Senior Registrar in Obstetrics and Gynaecology at Liverpool Women's Hospital, L8 7SS

Mr S Veck is Educational Coordinator at Surgical Technology, Newbury Road, Andover, Hampshire SP10 4DR

Dr C Nelson-Piercy is Consultant Physician at St Thomas' Hospital & Whipps Cross Hospital, London

Dr A Sultan is Senior Registrar in the Department of Obstetrics and Gynaecology, St George's Hospital, London SW17 OQT

Dr AK Monga is Consultant Gynaecologist at Princess Anne Hospital, Southampton

Dr SL Stanton is Consultant Gynaecologist in the Department of Obstetrics and Gynaecology, St George's Hospital, London SW17 OQT

Foreword

To write is to communicate. To communicate clearly is a great aspiration. To write clearly is the hardest task of all.

In the speciality of obstetrics and gynaecology, the practical art and the scientific core have to be blended and taught to trainees in a compact and clear way, in order to allow assimilation of an increasing technological area founded on a long and spirited tradition. The new learn from the old and the old learn from new advances in theory and applied practice. This book has attempted to blend the essential core knowledge, with its scientific, and often diverse background, thanks to a team of expert authors whose experience is invaluable and whose commitment to teaching is praiseworthy. My gratitude to the teachers and their efforts to communicate clearly is greatly appreciated.

Roy G Farquharson

1 Fetal biophysical profile scoring

SA Walkinshaw

Assessment of real-time ultrasound fetal biophysical variables has a limited role in the management of selected high-risk pregnancies. Composite biophysical scores remain inadequately studied and are of unproven value as a first-line test.

Fetal biophysical scoring, as developed by Manning *et al* (1980), has gained widespread acceptance as an integral part of antepartum fetal surveillance of high-risk pregnancies. The use of multiple ultrasound variables arose in part from dissatisfaction with the high false-positive rates associated with conventional monitoring using cardiotocography (Thacker and Berkelman, 1986) and in part from evaluation of other parameters such as liquor volume and fetal movement (Pearson and Weaver, 1976; Manning *et al*, 1981). It was hoped that more integrated strategies would both improve identification of the healthy fetus and more accurately separate out the sick fetus.

The main system used is that of Manning *et al* (1980) shown in its current form in Table 1, with clinical management being determined by the overall score. One other scoring system is used in some centres, with variables being graded 0, 1 or 2 and placental grading being included as a sixth parameter (Vintzileos *et al*, 1983).

Table 1. Biophysical profile scoring system A

Biophysical variable	Normal (score = 2)	Abnormal (score = 0)
Fetal breathing movements (FBM)	At least one episode of FBM of at least 30 seconds duration in 30 minutes observation	Absent FBM or no episode of >30 seconds in 30 minutes
Gross body movements	At least three discrete body/limb movements in 30 minutes (episodes of active continuous movement considered as single movement)	Two or fewer episodes of body/limb movements in 30 minutes
Fetal tone	At least one episode of active extension with return to flexion of fetal limb(s) or trunk. Opening and closing of hand considered normal tone	Either slow extension, with return to partial flexion, or movement of limb in full extension. Fetal movement absent
Reactive fetal heart rate (FHR)	At least two episodes of FHR acceleration of >15 beats/min and of at least 15 seconds duration associated with fetal movement in 30 minutes	Less than two episodes of acceleration of FHR or acceleration of >15 beats/min in 30 minutes
Qualitative amniotic fluid (AF) volume	At least one pocket of AF that measures at least 2 cm in two perpendicular planes	Either no AF pockets or a pocket <2 cm in two perpendicular planes

Score 8–10 (liquor normal) — normal score, Score 6 — equivocal; repeat within 24 hours, Score 8 (abnormal liquor) 0–4 — abnormal score; deliver if mature
from Manning *et al* (1980)

Underlying physiology

The application of biophysical scoring to obstetric pathology must include some understanding of the physiology of the parameters being used and the response of those variables to hypoxaemia and acidaemia. Fetal breathing, fetal body movement, fetal heart rate variability, and movement-associated heart rate accelerations all vary with the stage of gestation (Patrick *et al*, 1980, 1982; Natale *et al*, 1984; Gagnon *et al*, 1987). Some parameters exhibit cyclical patterns across a 24-hour period and are also subject to considerable influence by maternal factors. The potential effect of gestational age on the inter- pretation of biophysical scoring is seen in Table 2. The final variable, ie. amniotic fluid volume, is also dynamic, with marked changes occurring throughout gestation (Brace and Wolf, 1989).

Interpretation of a biophysical score in a particular clinical situation, therefore, requires consideration of the stage of gestation, time of day and a number of maternal factors. It also requires consideration of the implications of abnormalities in individual biophysical parameters.

The premise is that hypoxaemia results in depression of biophysical activities. Experimental evidence demonstrates reduction or cessation of fetal breathing activity and fetal movements (Boddy *et al*, 1974; Natale *et al*, 1981) and reduction in fetal heart rate reactivity (Visser *et al*, 1990) associated with fetal hypoxaemia. It has been suggested that the response to hypoxaemia varies, with some parameters being more sensitive than others (Vintzileos *et al*, 1983). There is human evidence to support such a concept, both from umbilical blood at delivery (Vintzileos *et al*, 1991) and from cordocentesis samples (Ribbert *et al*, 1990). From these studies it appears that loss of fetal breathing movement and of fetal heart rate variability are the most sensitive indices of hypoxaemia and acidaemia, with loss of fetal body movement occurring in more severe compromise. Loss of fetal muscle tone is a very late, virtually terminal phenomenon.

Reduction in amniotic fluid volume is regarded as a more chronic response to asphyxial stress. Recent work on the human fetus using pulsed and colour flow Doppler ultrasound appear to confirm animal studies demonstrating a redistribution of cardiac output and reduction in renal perfusion in the presence of hypoxaemia (Wladimiroff *et al*, 1987; Vyas *et al*, 1989).

Clinical role of biophysical profile scoring

The initial prospective studies of biophysical profile (BPP) scoring (Manning *et al*, 1980; Platt *et al*, 1983; Vintzileos *et al*, 1983) appeared to show improvement in false-positive rates over single parameter testing, although prediction of the healthy fetus was not improved using multiple tests. Randomised controlled studies comparing the non-stress test with the BPP (Manning *et al*, 1984; Platt *et al*, 1985) also suggested little improvement in the prediction of normality, but small improvements in the prediction of abnormality. Since then large interventional studies have been reported (Baskett *et al*, 1987; Manning *et al*, 1987; Vintzileos *et al*, 1987a). Excluding malformation, the risk of intrauterine death within 1 week of a normal profile appears to be 0.07%. However, false-positive prediction of perinatal mortality and morbidity remains high, with positive predictive values for indicators of fetal distress in the range of only 17% to 40% (Manning *et al*, 1990b).

How then should we use this method of fetal monitoring in practice? Large studies of high-risk populations tell us little about how to approach a particular pregnancy with a clearly defined pathology such as a fetus with suspected growth retardation.

Table 2. Effect of gestational age on fetal biophysical activity			
Gestation (weeks)	Maximum apnoea (min)	Maximum inactivity (min)	Percentage time in 1 hour less than 2 heart rate accelerations (> 15 bpm for 15 s)
26–28	14	24	65
30–31	68	75	2.7
34–35	108	75	2.7

Suspected growth retardation

The growth-retarded fetus would appear to be well suited to monitoring using biophysical parameters. Of all fetuses with scores of four or less, 40% were growth retarded (Manning *et al*, 1987), and where the score was zero, all intrauterine deaths, excluding anomaly and alloimmunisation, and over 80% of live-born infants were growth retarded (Manning *et al*, 1990a).

Nevertheless, as an individual group such pregnancies have been poorly studied. Suspected intrauterine growth retarded (IUGR) fetuses were excluded from one of the two randomised studies (Manning *et al*, 1984). Our own studies (Walkinshaw *et al*, 1992) suggest that amniotic fluid volume and cardiotocography are as effective as BPP scoring (Table 3). The addition of fetal breathing, should one of the original parameters be abnormal, improves the false-positive rate. Such a graded approach to monitoring is supported by other studies (Vintzileos *et al*, 1987a; Mills *et al*, 1990).

Table 3. Prediction of acidosis in a small-for-gestational-age (SGA) fetus				
	Sensitivity (%)	Specificity (%)	Predictive value positive	Predictive value negative
NST	19	88	0.28	0.82
AFV	31	83	0.31	0.83
NST + FBM	42	66	0.23	0.83
NST + AFV + FBM	31	87	0.36	0.84
BPP	42	78	0.32	0.83

NST=non-stress test, AFV=amniotic fluid volume, FBM=fetal breathing movements, BPP=biophysical profile
From Walkinshaw *et al*, 1992

Prolonged pregnancy

These pregnancies also fit the concept of gradual hypoxaemia due to placental insufficiency, and biophysical assessment would appear ideal. As a group these are better studied. Although claims have been made regarding the superiority of BPP scoring (Johnson *et al*, 1986), detailed analysis of most studies shows little advantage in positive predictive value of the BPP over cardiotocography or amniotic fluid volume alone, or over a combination of these methods (Walkinshaw, 1992). Therefore, although biophysical monitoring may be useful, BPP scoring is not.

Other specific pregnancy complications

Sudden unexpected fetal death is still a feared complication of pregnancy in the diabetic mother. Although the precise mode of death remains unclear, there is evidence that it may be hypoxaemic in nature. A number of studies have examined the use of the BPP in diabetic pregnancies (Golde *et al*, 1984; Dicker *et al*, 1988; Johnson *et al*, 1988) but none contained any such deaths. It is therefore difficult to be certain that the BPP is as reassuring as is claimed. The three diabetic still-births reported by Manning *et al* (1985) had a BPP score that was within 1 week of a normal score. Prediction of morbidity is poor in all studies. No comparative trials of the BPP against any other form of monitoring have been performed, and the advantage of the BPP in diabetic pregnancies is unsubstantiated.

Alloimmunised pregnancies make up a small proportion of tested pregnancies in most studies but there are few data to suggest that biophysical monitoring adds to the management of these pregnancies. Preliminary studies in twin pregnancies suggest a possible role for biophysical monitoring (Lodeiro *et al*, 1986; Baskett, 1989) with relatively better prediction of mortality and morbidity by such assessment. This may be because maternal variables and external stimuli that may affect biophysical activities are identical for each fetus. Thus differences in scores may be highly significant.

Pregnancies with preterm premature rupture of the membranes have been extensively assessed using the profile of Vintzileos *et al* (1983). Profile monitoring may predict fetal infection (Vintzileos *et al*, 1986) and its use on a daily basis coupled with prompt intervention may reduce the incidence of neonatal sepsis (Vintzileos *et al*, 1987b). Whether full scoring is needed or whether fetal breathing and cardioto-cography would be equally effective remains untested.

The future of biophysical monitoring

Despite extensive experience with this form of fetal surveillance, its precise role remains unclear. There seems little ground for its use as a routine or front-line test of fetal well-being. Nevertheless, there is no doubt that observable biophysical activities in the human fetus are influenced by hypoxaemia. From much published work a consistent theme is that negative predictive values are rarely significantly altered by multiple testing if one or two are normal. The situation in which biophysical testing may be of value is where one monitoring parameter is abnormal. The use of profile scoring, both as a back-up system and as a reminder that fetal surveillance should be as extensive as possible, will reduce unnecessary and ill-advised intervention.

Consideration must also be given as to whether BPP scoring should continue in its present form. It is now over a decade since its initial derivation. Both the definitions of normal and abnormal parameters and that of test duration need to be questioned, especially with regard to gestational age. The definition of abnormal liquor volume must be related to gestational age and to alternative methods of volume assessment such as the amniotic fluid index. The equal weighting of all parameters is no longer tenable, and has already been partially abandoned by many groups (Manning *et al*, 1990c). The value of continuing to include fetal tone, whose absence is largely a terminal event, must be in doubt.

Finally we must identify those obstetric pathologies where such monitoring is considered to be of value, and abandon its use as a 'catch-all' test. It may then be possible to assess the value of combinations of dynamic ultrasound variables and cardiotocography to fetal biophysical monitoring in well-conducted clinical trials, which to date, has not been addressed (Mohide and Kierse, 1989).

Key points

- There is a cyclical pattern to most fetal biophysical activities. These patterns and the activities themselves alter with gestational age.
- The sensitivity of different biophysical variables to hypoxaemia is not constant. This may affect predictive ability.
- Use of biophysical profile scoring may reduce unnecessary intervention based on a single abnormal test.
- Use of biophysical profile scoring should be limited to those high-risk conditions where it is of proven value.

References

Baskett TF (1989) Fetal biophysical profile. In: Studd J, ed. *Progress in Obstetrics and Gynaecology*. Churchill Livingstone, Edinburgh: vol 7: 145–60

Baskett TF, Allen AC, Gray JH, Young DC, Young LM (1987) Fetal biophysical profile and perinatal death. *Obstet Gynecol* **70**: 357–9

Brace RA, Wolf EJ (1989) Normal amniotic fluid volume changes throughout pregnancy. *Am J Obstet Gynecol* **161**: 382–8

Boddy K, Dawes GS, Fisher R *et al* (1974) Fetal respiratory movements, electro-cortical and cardiovascular responses to hypoxaemia and hypercapnia in sleep. *J Physiol* **243**: 599–606

Dicker D, Feldberg D, Yeshaya A, Peleg D, Karp M, Goldman JA (1988) Fetal surveillance in insulin-dependent diabetic pregnancy: Predictive value of the biophysical profile. *Am J Obstet Gynecol* **159**: 800–4

Gagnon R, Campbell K, Hunse C, Patrick J (1987) Patterns of human fetal heart rate accelerations from 26 weeks to term. *Am J Obstet Gynecol* **157**: 743–8

Golde SH, Montoro M, Good-Anderson B *et al* (1984) The role of nonstress tests, fetal biophysical profile, and contraction stress tests in the outpatient management of insulin-requiring diabetic pregnancies. *Am J Obstet Gynecol* **148**: 269–73

Johnson JM, Harman CR, Lange IR, Manning FA (1986) Biophysical profile scoring in the management of the postterm pregnancy; an analysis of 307 patients. *Am J Obstet Gynecol* **154**: 269–73

Johnson JM, Lange IR, Harman CR, Torchia MG, Manning FA (1988) Biophysical profile scoring in the management of the diabetic pregnancy. *Obstet Gynecol* **72**: 841–6

Lodeiro JG, Vintzileos AM, Feinstein SJ, Campbell WA, Nochimson DJ (1986) Fetal biophysical profile in twin gestations. *Obstet Gynecol* **67**: 824–7

Manning FA, Platt LD, Sipos L (1980) Antepartum fetal evaluation : development of a fetal biophysical profile. *Am J Obstet Gynecol* **136**: 787–95

Manning FA, Hill LM, Platt LD (1981) Quantitative amniotic fluid volume determination by ultrasound: antepartum detection of intrauterine growth retardation. *Am J Obstet Gynecol* **139**: 254–8

Manning FA, Lange IR, Morrison I, Harman CR (1984) Fetal biophysical profile and the nonstress test: a comparative trial. *Obstet Gynecol* **64**: 326–31

Manning FA, Morrison I, Lange IR, Harman CR, Chamberlain PF (1985) Fetal assessment based on fetal biophysical profile scoring: experience in 12 620 referred high-risk pregnancies. I. Perinatal mortality by frequency and etiology. *Am J Obstet Gynecol* **151**: 343–50

Manning FA, Morrison I, Harman CR, Lange IR, Menticoglou S (1987) Fetal assessment based on fetal biophysical profile scoring: experience in 19 221 referred high-risk pregnancies. II. An analysis of false negative fetal deaths. *Am J Obstet Gynecol* **157**: 880–4

Manning FA, Harman CR, Morrison IR, Menticoglou SM (1990a) Fetal assessment based on fetal biophysical profile scoring. III. Positive predictive accuracy of the very abnormal test (biophysical profile score = 0). *Am J Obstet Gynecol* **162**: 398–402

Manning FA, Harman CR, Morrison I, Menticoglou SM, Lange IR, Johnson JM (1990b) Fetal assessment based on fetal biophysical profile scoring. IV. An analysis of perinatal mortality and morbidity. *Am J Obstet Gynecol* **162**: 703–9

Manning FA, Morrison IR, Harman CR, Menticoglou SM (1990c) The abnormal fetal biophysical profile score. V. Predictive accuracy according to score composition. *Am J Obstet Gynecol* **162**: 918–27

Mills MS, James DK, Slade S (1990) Two-tier approach to biophysical assessment of the fetus. *Am J Obstet Gynecol* **163**: 12–16

Mohide P, Kierse M (1989) In: Chalmers I, Enkin M, Kierse MJNC, eds. *Effective Care in Pregnancy and Childbirth. Vol 1. Pregnancy.* Oxford University Press, Oxford: 477–92

Natale R, Clewlow F, Dawes GS (1981) Measurement of fetal forelimb movement in the lamb in utero. *Am J Obstet Gynecol* **140**: 545–51

Natale R, Nasello C, Turliuk R (1984) The relationship between movements and accelerations in fetal heart rate at twenty-four to thirty-two weeks' gestation. *Am J Obstet Gynecol* **148**: 591–5

Patrick J, Campbell K, Carmichael L *et al* (1980) A definition of human fetal apnea and the distribution of fetal apneic intervals in the last ten weeks of pregnancy. *Am J Obstet Gynecol* **136**: 471–7

Patrick J, Campbell K, Carmichael L *et al* (1982) Patterns of gross fetal body movements over 24-hour observation intervals in the last ten weeks of pregnancy. *Am J Obstet Gynecol* **142**: 363–71

Pearson JF, Weaver JB (1976) Fetal activity and fetal well-being: an evaluation. *Br Med J* **i**: 1305–7

Platt LD, Eglinton GS, Sipos L, Broussard PM, Paul RH (1983) Further experience with the fetal biophysical profile. *Obstet Gynecol* **61**: 480–5

Platt LD, Walla C, Paul RH, Trujillo ME, Loesser CV, Jacobs ND, Broussard PM (1985) A prospective trial of the fetal biophysical profile versus the nonstress test in the management of high-risk pregnancies. *Am J Obstet Gynecol* **153**: 624–33

Ribbert LSM, Snijders RJM, Nicolaides KH, Visser GHA (1990) Relationship of fetal biophysical profile and blood gas values at cordocentesis in severely growth-retarded fetuses. *Am J Obstet Gynecol* **163**: 569–71

Thacker SB, Berkelman RL (1986) Assessing the diagnostic accuracy and efficacy of selected antepartum fetal surveillance techniques. *Obstet Gynecol Surv* **41**: 121–41

Vintzileos AM, Campbell WA, Ingardia CJ, Nochimson DJ (1983) The fetal biophysical profile and its predictive value. *Obstet Gynecol* **62**: 271–8

Vintzileos AM, Campbell WA, Nochimson DJ, Weinbaum PJ (1986) Fetal biophysical profile versus amniocentesis in predicting infection in preterm premature rupture of the membranes. *Obstet Gynecol* **68**: 488–94

Vintzileos AM, Campbell WA, Nochimson DJ, Weinbaum PJ (1987a) The use and misuse of the fetal biophysical profile. *Am J Obstet Gynecol* **156**: 527–33

Vintzileos AM, Bors-Koefoed R, Pelegano JF *et al* (1987b) The use of the fetal biophysical profile improves pregnancy outcome in premature rupture of the membranes. *Am J Obstet Gynecol* **157**: 236–40

Vintzileos AM, Fleming AD, Scorza WE *et al* (1991) Relationship between fetal biophysical activities and umbilical cord blood gas values. *Am J Obstet Gynecol* **165**: 707–13

Visser GA, Sadovsky G, Nicolaides KH (1990) Antepartum heart rate patterns in small-for-gestational-age third trimester fetuses: correlations with blood gas values obtained at cordocentesis. *Am J Obstet Gynecol* **162**: 698–703

Vyas S, Nicolaides KH, Campbell S (1989) Renal artery flow-velocity waveforms in normal and hypoxemic fetuses. *Am J Obstet Gynecol* **161**: 168–72

Walkinshaw SA (1992) Biophysical profile scoring — a critical review. In: Neilson J, Chambers S, eds. *Obstetric Ultrasound.* Oxford Univesity Press, Oxford: 1

Walkinshaw SA, Cameron H, McPhail S, Robson S (1992) The prediction of fetal compromise and acidosis by biophysical profile scoring in the small for gestational age fetus. *J Perinat Med* **20** (3): 227–232

Wladimiroff JW, Winjgaard JAGW, Degani S, Noordam J, van Eyck J, Tonge HM (1987) Cerebral and umbilical arterial flow velocity waveforms in normal and growth retarded pregnancies. *Obstet Gynecol* **69**: 705–9

2 MRCOG Part Two: facing the *viva*

RG Farquharson

The viva examination has two parts: the clinical and the viva voce. This chapter presents practical advice on how best to approach what is rightly felt by many to be the most hazardous part of the MRCOG Part Two examination.

The *viva* examination forms an integral part of the Part Two MRCOG examination. Most candidates rightly believe this to be the most hazardous part of the examination. Certainly, many who fail do so here. At present, only candidates who have passed the written part are allowed to take the *viva*. Thus, candidates at least have the confidence of knowing that they have already passed the written part.

The *viva* has two parts: one clinical and one *viva voce* examination. These are usually taken on the same day at different hospitals in major cities in the UK. The first is an assessment of the candidate's ability to take a comprehensive history from a patient and present his or her findings to the examiners. Thereafter, a shorter discussion follows regarding the investigation and treatment of the patient's condition. This is a reasonably straightforward part in which all candidates should do well.

The second examination is more a discussion forum where controversial issues can be aired and the candidate's ability to analyse as well as criticise is assessed in an examination atmosphere. It is at this stage that all candidates realise the importance of participating in mock *vivas* organised either by the local district tutor of the RCOG or by consultants in their hospital. Many Part Two courses offer a video facility so candidates can assess their own performance. The value of mock *vivas* cannot be over-emphasised.

The college examiners want to hear all you have to offer. They despair when they have to seek answers as if drawing blood from a stone. You should make no mono-syllabic answers unless a yes/no response is demanded. Do not look for the obtuse or the obscure angle of a particular item of discussion. Examiners are interested in common sense applied to clinical practice. They wish to know the depth of your knowledge or experience on a particular matter. If you are in doubt about the question then it is only proper to ask for more details. This will help, not only to prolong and deepen discussion, but also to arrive at a suitable endpoint at which the examiners feel confident about your ability and clinical competence.

If your mind goes blank think of the last clinically relevant case you encountered and explain the process which led to the decision. Be critical, to show the examiners that you can analyse problems and can apply good clinical practice to a difficult situation. Start with simple answers; often the obvious is being asked. If an examiner wishes you to expand on a certain point, he or she will ask you *during* the development of the question.

MRCOG book

Remember, the *viva* is an assessment of your competence to practise and not your knowledge of the small print. Know your MRCOG book well before the examination and refresh your memory beforehand, so that if a particular case is taken from the book for discussion you will be familiar with its contents. When it gets down to the nitty-gritty be prepared to defend your decisions clearly and concisely. Although the examiner may see a situation differently from you, it is just a difference of opinion and not necessarily correct. A difference of opinion will not fail you if you can defend yourself adequately. It is best to avoid repeating a particular author's work parrot-fashion and you should always be prepared to give a broader view in the presentation of a subject. This shows that you are enlightened and are willing to appreciate other views on a similar matter.

A historical perspective is as useful as a knowledge of the cutting edge of a particular area of research. It is always essential to know the background to a problem and to be aware of what previous obstetricians and gynaecologists thought on the subject before arriving at a conclusion on a clinical case type or investigation. Do not be too anxious to list causes or differential diagnoses, but introduce each with a reason for mentioning them.

3 Management of an abnormal smear

W Prendiville

While large loop excision of the transformation zone is not a difficult technique, important principles must be considered to avoid complications. This chapter presents practical advice to deal with most circumstances that may arise. Postoperative protocols and efficacy are also covered.

In this chapter emphasis is given to the practical problems associated with large loop excision of the transformation zone (LLETZ).

Equipment

A comfortable colposcopy couch is essential for a colposcopic examination. One that allows the colposcopist to elevate and tilt the couch offers a great advantage, as it will spare the examiner's back; it is important to be comfortable while performing these procedures if one is proposing to do any number of them.

A number of very good colposcopes are available. In choosing one, the ergonomics of the machine are probably as important as the optics. Also, it is important to ensure that the colposcope has a low enough magnification to view the entire cervix in one field. The focal length should be at least 300 mm, otherwise it is not easy to place the loop electrode 'pencil' between the colposcope and the patient. A choice of speculae will be necessary and the range should include some that are small enough to insert through a nulliparous introitus and others that are large enough to visualise the largest cervix through the most capacious vagina.

Sometimes, even when using a large speculum, the lateral vaginal walls may fall medially, thereby obscuring part or all of the cervix. In these circumstances, a condom (with its end cut off) is a useful means of holding back the vagina walls. A cheaper alternative is the finger of a latex glove.

Analgesia

LLETZ and indeed small loop biopsies require an anaesthetic. Very occasionally a patient will have difficulty accommodating even a speculum examination and in this case it is preferable to perform colposcopy and, where necessary, LLETZ under general anaesthesia. Circumstances which *may* warrant a general anaesthetic include:

1. A very atropic cervix that is almost flush with the vaginal wall.
2. A very large transformation zone (TZ) that extends to, or is close to, the vaginal epithelium.
3. Excessive difficulty in achieving comfortable access to the cervix.

However, it is possible to remove a cone-shaped biopsy using LLETZ. The geography and dimension of the TZ need no longer dictate general anaesthesia. For most women it is feasible to remove the TZ under local anaesthesia.

There are a number of alternative approaches to achieving sufficient insensitivity of the cervical TZ in order to perform LLETZ. Paracervical block has enjoyed fairly fickle popularity for several minor gynaecological procedures, ranging from intrauterine contraceptive device insertion (and removal) to hysteroscopy and dilatation and curettage. However, it is not always effective.

Local infiltration, on the other hand, is virtually guaranteed to achieve complete insensitivity of the epithelium to be resected. Lignocaine, with or without adrenaline, is widely used; however, the very rapid serum uptake of adrenaline following infiltration is intimidating (Low *et al*, 1984). Citanest with octapressin is probably a wiser choice, given its lack of cardiotoxity. Infiltration may be achieved using an ordinary needle and syringe; better, though, is the dental syringe system. The vials slip easily in and out of the cartridge cyclinder without one having to change the needle. There are a number of needle sizes, the 27g probably being the most appropriate for the cervix. The relative narrowness of the dental syringe does not preclude adequate visibility of the cervix while in use, which may be a problem if ordinary syringes are used. The vials each contain 2.2 ml, so several may be necessary to completely block sensation underneath and around the TZ. It is preferable to overestimate rather than underestimate the volume necessary. Initially the injection should be slow and just subepithelial. Subsequent deeper infiltration may then be performed almost unnoticed by the patient.

The technique of LLETZ

LLETZ is not a technically demanding skill, particularly if the cervix is clean, non-pregnant or non-puerperal, well infiltrated with local anaesthetic, and reveals a fully visible small ectocervical TZ. A warm, relaxed and informed patient completes the ideal conditions for LLETZ.

Following a thorough colposcopic examination, the following steps should be taken before approaching the cervix with a loop:

1. Attach the diathermy plate to the patient.
2. Apply suction to the speculum's suction tube.
3. Choose and insert a loop of appropriate dimensions into the diathermy pencil.
4. Focus the colposcope using a low magnification such that the entire TZ is visible within one field of view.
5. Select the appropriate power setting for both the cutting and coagulation modes and choose a blend ratio.

With the activating button depressed (and blended diathermy chosen), the loop is applied to the cervix 5 mm outside the lateral margins of the TZ. It is then brought slowly underneath the TZ before exiting at approximately the same distance from the contralateral TZ margin. The procedure is illustrated diagrammatically in Figure 1.

While performing the procedure, one should try to be conscious of the depth of the loop within the cervix. Anderson and Hartley (1980) clearly demonstrated that dysplastic epithelium may be present in the TZ up to 6 mm below the surface epithelium. The intention at LLETZ should be to remove the same amount of tissue, and no more, than would a destructive method, which is 8–10 mm below the TZ surface epithelium. Of course, the TZ does not have a flat surface; rather it is both convex and concave. One's choice of loop or loops should take into account the contour of the TZ such that the depth of tissue excised is at least 8 mm throughout.

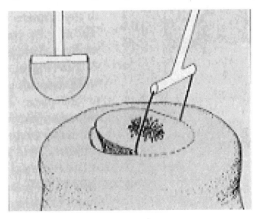

Figure 1. Diagrammatic representation of large loop excision of the transformation

Selection of instrumentation and power settings

Although LLETZ is not a difficult technique, it is quite easy to make it so. Three basic principles deserve consideration:

1. LLETZ should only be performed following a competent colposcopic examination by an experienced colposcopist; it is not a procedure for the occasional colposcopist.

2. The intention of LLETZ should be to remove the entire TZ. An adequate margin of normal epithelium should surround the dysplastic process. The squamocolumnar junction should be clearly evident to the pathologist when he/she examines each section of the excised specimen.

3. LLETZ should inflict the minimal amount of artefactual damage to the biopsy specimen that has been removed and to the cervical wound.

In order to achieve these, an appreciation of the anatomy of the TZ and the principles of electrosurgery are crucial (Billings and McLucas, 1992), the most important being the difference between fulguration and desiccation (Figure 2).

In practice, fulgurative electrosurgery occurs most completely when the wire is spaced 1 mm or so from the tissue to be resected. This is not easy; few of us are able to appreciate this distance visually let alone have the digital dexterity and steadiness of hand to keep the wire consistently spaced above the tissue. Furthermore, for the

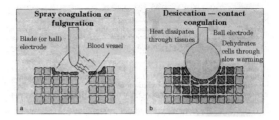

Figure 2. Fulguration (a) and desiccation (b)

most part the wire is not visible to the operator. In order to maximise the degree of fulguration and minimise the degree of desiccation two precepts should be borne in mind:

1. Choose power output levels that will maintain a voltage of >200V throughout the procedure.

2. Allow the current to spark ahead of the wire. If the wire is passed slowly through the cervical tissue it will create its own 'steam envelope'. The wire will thus (almost) never be in actual contact with the cells and a fulgurative cutting and coagulative effect will ensue. If the wire is 'pushed' through the tissue to any degree it will be pressed against the tissue ahead of it and, inevitably, will inflict desiccative artefactual damage. The wire should never need to be pushed (or pulled) through the tissue so that its shape or angle of inclination is altered in any way, ie. the wire should not bend. A slow but steady hand is the key to a smooth, clean and dry passage through the cervical tissue.

Common circumstances

Figures 3–13 depict the most common circumstances encountered in a busy colposcopy service. These examples are not exhaustive; by modifying these choices, however, a colposcopist should be able to perform LLETZ in any circumstance that may arise.

Figure 3 illustrates perhaps the most common circumstance, where the entire transformation zone is easily visualised because it lies on the ectocervix, or where its upper limit lies <5 mm inside the endocervical canal. Also, it is medium sized, which is here defined as a TZ that does not exceed 18 mm in any diameter. In these circumstances the TZ may be conveniently excised using a medium (white) loop with dimensions 20 mm (width) x 15 mm (depth). This loop will excise this type of TZ in one sweep and in one piece. The all-important squamocolumnar junction will be well clear of

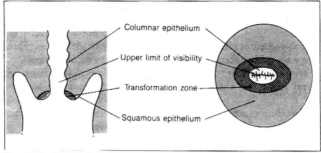

Figure 3. The fully visible and ectocervical transformation zone

the diathermy excision margin. This procedure is illustrated in Figure 4.

For those colposcopists who are early in their LLETZ learning curve, an alternative means of dealing with the TZ is to excise it in two pieces using smaller loops. This is an entirely reasonable option and some colposcopists will choose to continue to practise in this way; Figure 5 portrays this

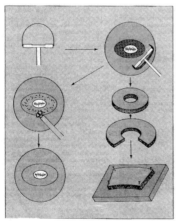

Figure 4. Large loop excision of the transformation zone: single sweep of the ectocervical transformation zone

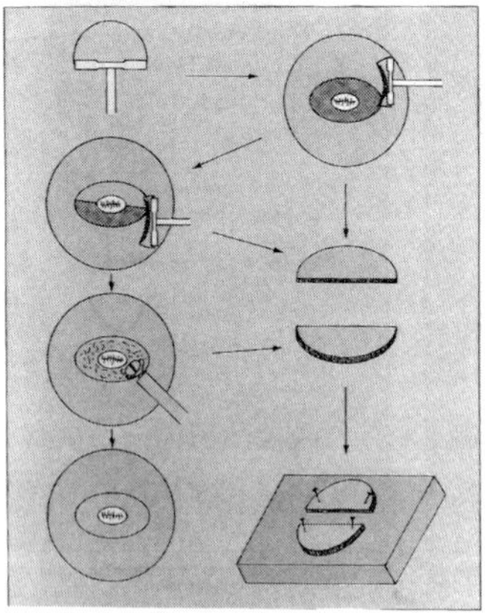

Figure 5. Large loop excision of the transformation zone: the two-piece technique

22

approach. A disadvantage is that by transecting the TZ in two pieces, one may damage the squamocolumnar junction.

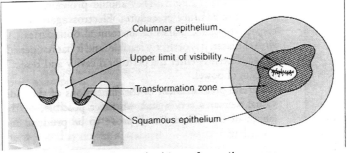

Columnar epithelium

Upper limit of visibility

Transformation zone

Squamous epithelium

Figure 6. A wide ectocervical transformation zone

Figure 6 represents a relatively frequent situation where the TZ is just too wide to be excised in a single sweep with the medium (20 x 15 mm) loop. In the absence of a suspicion of microinvasion or glandular disease, several options are available. It is not helpful to be dogmatic about which of these options is the best for a particular cervix or an individual surgeon. They are (in order of the author's preference):

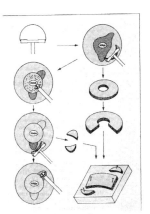

Figure 7. Large loop excision of the transformation zone: the wide transformation zone, example a

1. Remove the central portion of the TZ in one sweep of a medium loop (20 x 15 mm), including the squamo-columnar junction. Remove the peripheral TZ separately as one or more pieces with one or more passes of the medium or a smaller loop (Figure 7).

2. Remove the TZ in two pieces with the medium loop.

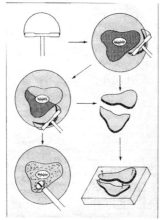

Figure 8. Large loop excision of the transformation zone: the wide transformation zone, example b

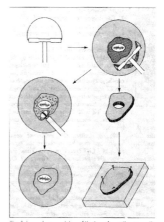

Figure 9. Large loop excision of the transformation zone: the wide transformation zone, example c

Usually the anterior cervical lip TZ is excised first and the posterior position second (Figure 8).

3.   Remove the entire TZ with one sweep using a larger/ wider loop (Figure 9).

The type of TZ illustrated in Figure 10 may not be visible at the first colposcopic assessment, but with the aid of endogenous and exogenous oestrogen it may become so. When faced with such a TZ, several options are available (ranked in order of the author's preference):

1.   Excise the entire TZ with one sweep of a long loop (20 x 20 mm) (Figure 11).

2.   Excise the ectocervical TZ using the usual (white) medium loop in one piece, then subsequently excise the remaining endocervical part of the TZ using a small to medium (green) loop (Figure 12).

3.   Fashion a cone biopsy using a 1 cm long straight wire as a knife (Figure 13).

Other circumstances that may be accommodated by LLETZ include:

1. An incompletely visible TZ.
2. The 'original' or congenital TZ.
3. A suspicion of microinvasive disease.
4. A suspicion of glandular abnormality.

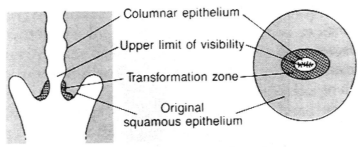

Figure 10. The largely endocervical transformation zone

An incompletely visible TZ

Where the TZ extends beyond view up the endocervical canal, it is necessary to perform a cone biopsy. The length of the cone biopsy may be gauged by determining the length of the TZ within the endocervical canal using a microcolpo-hysteroscope and Watermans blue ink. Alternatively, one may presume that the TZ is 20–25 mm up the canal and perform a conization of at least this length.

Having decided the length of cone biopsy, one then has to choose the technique of LLETZ cone method. These are essentially those detailed in Figures 11–13. Of course, where the cone biopsy is removed using the single loop technique described in Figure 13, a loop of appropriate dimensions must be utilised. The potential for not achieving a satisfactory LLETZ cone will increase with the length of the TZ in the endocervical canal and decrease with the experience of the colposcopist.

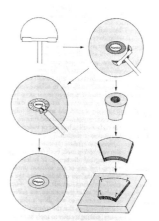

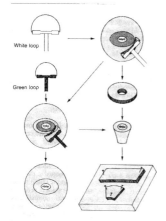

Figure 11. Large loop excision of the transformation zone: cone, example a

Figure 12. Large loop excision of the transformation zone: cone, example b

Large LLETZ cones taken with a single sweep of a large loop should not be undertaken lightly or by a colposcopist who has not had considerable experience with LLETZ. They should probably not be undertaken as office procedures. Electrosurgery has no respect for tissue planes or anatomical boundaries. As with the laser, it is perfectly feasible (and it has happened) to inadvertently enter the peritoneal cavity and resect a portion of bowel.

Careful preassessment of the dimensions of the individual woman's cervix and, wherever possible, of the length of the TZ itself will prove to be prudent and rewarding.

Original or congenital TZ

Approximately 4% of women will have a TZ that extends onto the vaginal epithelium. This in itself is not pathological, but it poses particular management problems when such a woman has an abnormal smear. This may be the only situation where it is reasonable to selectively remove the apparently dysplastic epithelium, but not the entire TZ. The author favours two therapeutic alternatives.

First, one may remove the apparent area of dysplasia within the TZ (when it is confined to the usual cervical epithelium) using LLETZ. The peripheral TZ may be monitored by cytological and colposcopic follow-up. The normality of the peripheral (vaginal) aspects of the TZ may be obvious on colposcopic examination, but where there is doubt, directed biopsies should be taken.

Second, the peripheral cervical and vaginal parts of the TZ may be destroyed using fulgurative rollerball diathermy, and again the more central cervical TZ containing the dysplastic epithelium may be excised. An alternative to rollerball fulgurative diathermy would, of course, be laser evaporation.

Suspicion of invasive disease

Microinvasive or early invasive disease deserves special attention. If such a diagnosis is suspected, the TZ should be removed in one piece with generous disease-free margins. This will offer a patient the best possible histological assessment. Where a TZ is fully visible, it will usually be possible to achieve this using an appropriately sized loop. Where the TZ is not fully visible or if it is exceptionally large, it may be preferable to choose the straight wire as a knife and fashion a cone biopsy in the same way as one might previously have used a cold knife or laser beam (Figure 13). This technique takes longer and usually demands general anaesthesia.

Suspicion of glandular abnormality

Most (90%) glandular disease is situated within 10 mm of the squamocolumnar junction; it is not usually recognisable colpo- scopically. Where it is, or where a cervical smear has raised the suspicion, a general length of endocervical glandular epithelium should be included with the excised TZ. As with micro-invasive or early invasive disease, it is preferable to remove the biopsy in one piece. How this is achieved will depend on the dimensions and site of the TZ; the options described in Figures 11–13 will cover most such cases.

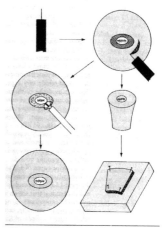

Post-LLETZ management of the cervix

Figure 13. Large loop excision of the transformation zone: cone, example c

The majority of post-LLETZ cervical wounds do not bleed excessively. The coagulative component of the blended diathermy will usually accommodate any vessels transected in the course of the procedure. Despite this, it has always been the author's practice to perform one of several prophylactic haemostatic procedures.

Several choices are available and all have been tried. Immediate post-LLETZ management options include:

1. Ball coagulation
2. Rollerball coagulation
3. Oxycel or other haemostatic gauze application
4. Packing of the wound with gauze soaked in ferric subsulphate
5. Packing of the wound with dry gauze
6. Silver nitrate
7. Ferric subsulphate application
8. Sultrin cream
9. No further intervention.

Probably the most widely used means of achieving complete

haemostasis is to 'cover' the wound with a very superficial application of coagulative diathermy using a ball end at about 30–40 W of output and selecting the pure coagulative modality on the electrosurgical unit. When using this method, one should dab the ball on and off the tissue as quickly as possible in order to avoid excessive artefactual damage caused by desiccating diathermy and to prevent the ball sticking to the wound.

A superior means of applying fulgurative and coagulative diathermy in order to seal the post-LLETZ wound is to employ a rollerball such as that shown in Figure 14. This rollerball incorporates a non-conductive rubber spacer

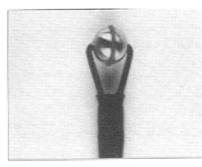

centrally, which helps to achieve a greater degree of fulguration. The rollerball rides over the surface of the wound much more quickly than the fixed ball and as a result achieves a dry surface with a very superficial layer of coagulation in a matter of moments. It is likely that this method will inflict less artefactual damage to the wound than the fixed ball. It is difficult to quantify the amount of fulgura- ting diathermy that should be applied. It should be sufficient to achieve complete haemostasis, but not so much as to inflict clinically important artefactual damage. With a dry wound, the amount of fulguration necessary is minimal and running over the surface with a ball end or rollerball can be achieved in seconds.

Figure 14. A rollerball diathermy electrode.

Ferric subsulphate (Monsel's solution) is also very widely used, both on its own and following ball diathermy. It is important not to spill any of the solution onto the vaginal epithelium or indeed onto the cervical epithelium outside of the wound. Leaving 20 ml of the solution in a galleypot for 48 hours or so will allow a degree of evaporation such that the solution becomes a paste, making it easier to apply but equally effective.

The other techniques listed in 1–9 are less popular and their efficacy needs to be evaluated by way of large randomised controlled trials.

The preceding discussion related to the routine prevention of bleeding by attempting to seal the wound. Where there is significant bleeding from the post-LLETZ wound, it will be due to an individual bleeding vessel. Three haemostatic techniques may be employed:

1. The coagulation output is turned up to 50 W and the ball end sited in the blood covering the wound. After a few seconds the blood will be coagulated and, thereafter, so will the bleeding vessel.

2. Excess blood is evacuated by sucking it away from the wound, thereby exposing the bleeding point which may then be conveniently coagulated.

3. The bleeding point is compressed by a small cotton tip bud and the surface of the wound is then dried with a cotton wool ball. By slowly rolling the cotton tip bud (or jumbo swab) off the bleeding point, it may be exposed and coagulated.

The last two techniques are superior to the first because much less power is necessary to effect haemostasis and therefore less artefactual damage is inflicted upon the wound. These techniques need to be performed under direct colposcopic vision. In this way, even quite large bleeding vessels may be isolated and dealt with. If this technique is followed it will rarely, if ever, be necessary to resort to general anaesthesia and suturing of the cervix in the face of persistent blood loss, even with a pregnant cervix.

Management of the biopsy

Although the majority of LLETZ specimens will be shallow and not involve the endocervical canal, from the pathologist's point of view these specimens may be considered in the same way as a cone biopsy. The logistics of processing small loop and LLETZ or cone biopsy specimens have been dealt with exhaustively in Cartier's (1984) atlas of colposcopy. The issue has also been dealt with more recently by Codling and Barry-Walsh (1992).

The clinician can greatly aid the pathologist by opening the biopsy before it is placed in formalin solution. Once in formalin, it is far more difficult to open and 'stretch out'. An open biopsy is of course easier to section serially than is a cone- or cylinder-shaped LLETZ specimen.

Opening the biopsy and pinning it to a cork pad before immersion in formalin takes only a few seconds of a colposcopist's (or his/her attendant nurse's) time and is well worth the effort. In so doing, one should be careful not to handle the tissue excessively to avoid dislodging any epithelium.

Management of the patient

Following LLETZ, a patient should avoid intercourse or vaginal tampons for approximately 4 weeks. Opinions vary as to the value of routine vaginal antibiotic cream (Sultrin, Metrogel) or oral antibiotics and neither advice has been tested in a randomised control trial. It is not uncommon to experience some slight bleeding per vaginam for a number of days, or even weeks, following LLETZ. If, however, this loss approaches that of normal menses, the patient should be examined again. Sometimes a single bleeding point will be evident which may conveniently be dealt with by diathermy coagulation under local anaesthesia. The more generalised ooze of blood associated with cervicitis is better dealt with by local and systemic antibiotics.

While there is no substitute for one-to-one counselling of patients, information hand-outs are a useful complementary way of reinforcing the details discussed at a patient's visit. As most patients only visit the clinic for colposcopic assessment and treatment, the preliminary and post-LLETZ interviews are important opportunities to counsel patients with regard to LLETZ, colposcopy and cervical intraepithelial neoplasia.

Efficacy of LLETZ

The first series of patients followed up for at least 12 months (Prendiville *et al*, 1989) achieved negative cytology and normal colposcopy rates of 97%. A single case of unsuspected microinvasion was revealed. Several authors have since reported the revelation of unsuspected microinvasion (Byrne and Saint Cassia, 1989; McIndoe *et al*, 1989; Phipps *et al*, 1989). Gunaskera *et al* (1990) published the first comparison of LLETZ with a destructive technique (laser). In their study the LLETZ patients had a lower risk of postoperative haemorrhage and discomfort. Operating time was reduced and there was no difference in the risk of recurrent abnormality. Wright and associates (1992) described a similar experience when comparing LLETZ with laser cone biopsies.

The number of published series reporting LLETZ is small (Prendiville and Cullimore, 1987; Prendiville *et al*, 1989; Bigrigg *et al*, 1990; Keijser *et al*, 1990; Luesley *et al*, 1990; Mor-Yosef *et al*, 1990; Whiteley and Olah, 1990; Murdoch *et al*, 1991; Wright *et al*, 1992), as is the length of patient follow-up in these series. However, the consistency between them would suggest that LLETZ is as efficacious as any of the destructive modalities. The occasional but consistent finding of unsuspected microinvasion is the most powerful argument for switching from a destructive method of treatment to LLETZ. Murdoch *et al's* (1991) large series of

1143 patients treated by LLETZ revealed 46 invasive carcinomas; 11 had not been suspected colposcopically or cytologically. The clinical experience of LLETZ has been comprehensively reviewed by Bigrigg (1992). Longer-term follow-up is awaited. Of particular interest will be the effect, if any, upon cervical dysfunction in terms of cervical stenosis, subfertility and cervical problems during labour.

Finally, there are a variety of post-LLETZ practices for management of the post-LLETZ cervical wound. Most practitioners use a simple ball end to cover the wound with coagulative diathermy in order to achieve and maintain a dry wound. Others use Monsel's solution or paste. Some pack the wound with dry or Monsel's solution-soaked gauze. Prophylactic antibiotics are used by a small proportion of practitioners.

There is a need for a large randomised controlled trial to compare these practices in order to determine which is the most effective and acceptable to the patient.

Key points

- Large loop excision of the transformation zone (LLETZ) should be avoided in women with evidence of cervicitis.
- LLETZ should always be performed under colposcopic guidance.
- LLETZ demands a competent colposcopic examination prior to the procedure.
- When performing LLETZ, aim to remove the entire transformation zone.
- Aim to inflict the minimum amount of artefactual damage by utilising a fulgurative rather than a desiccative electrosurgical technique.
- Audit of patients following treatment is essential.

Sincere gratitude is owed to Dr Rene Cartier for his help and advice with the develop-

ment of LLETZ. I wish to thank Fidelma Kavanagh for careful preparation of this article. The figures are reproduced by kind permission of Chapman and Hall, Mosby Year Book and the British Journal of Obstetrics and Gynaecology.

References

Anderson MC, Hartley RB (1980) Cervical crypt involvement by intraepithelial neoplasia. *Obstet Gynecol* **55**: 546–50

Bigrigg A (1992) Overview of clinical experience to date. In: Prendiville W, ed. *LLETZ: A Practical Guide*. Chapman and Hall, London

Bigrigg A, Codling BW, Pearson P (1990) Colposcopic diagnosis and treatment of cervical dysplasia at a single clinic visit. *Lancet* **ii**: 229–36

Billings G, McLucas B (1992) The principles of low voltage blended diathermy surgery. In: Prendiville W, ed. *LLETZ: A Practical Guide*. Chapman and Hall, London

Byrne PF, Saint Cassia LJ (1989) Occult cervical carcinoma revealed by large loop diathermy. *Lancet* **ii**: 807

Cartier R (1984) *Colposcopie Pratique*. 2nd edn. Laboratoire Cartier, Paris

Codling B, Barry-Walsh C (1992) Pathological processing and interpretation. In: Prendiville W, ed. *LLETZ: A Practical Guide*. Chapman and Hall, London

Gunaskera PC, Phipps JM, Lewis BV (1990) Large loop excision of the transformation zone (LLETZ) compared to carbon dioxide laser in the treatment of CIN: a superior mode of treatment. *Br J Obstet Gynaecol* **97**: 995–8

Keijser KCG, van der Zanden P, Schijt CPT (1990) Diathermy loop and CIN lesions. *J Exp Clin Cancer Res* **9**:1

Low JM, Harvey JT, Cooper GM, Prendiville W (1984) Plasma concentrations of catecholamines following adrenaline infiltration during gynaecological surgery. *Br J Anaesth* **56**: 849–53

Luesley DM, Cullimore J, Redman CWE (1990) Loop diathermy excision of the cervical transformation zone in patients with abnormal cervical smears. *Br Med J* **300**: 1690–3

McIndoe GAJ, Smith JR, Tidy JA *et al* (1989) Occult cervical carcinoma revealed by large loop diathermy. *Lancet* **ii**: 807

Mor-Yosef S, Lopes A, Pearson S, Monaghan JM (1990) Loop diathermy cone biopsy. *Obstet Gynecol* **75**: 884–6

Murdoch JB, Grimshaw JM, Monaghan SM (1991) Loop diathermy excision of the abnormal cervical transformation zone. *Int J Gynaecol Cancer* **1**: 105–11

Phipps JM, Gunasekera PC, Lewis BV (1989) Occult cervical carcinoma revealed by large loop diathermy. *Lancet* **ii**: 453

Prendiville W, Cullimore J (1987) Excision of the transformation zone using the low voltage diathermy (LVD) loop: A superior method of treatment. *Colposcopy Gynaecol Laser Surg* **3**: 225

Prendiville W, Cullimore J, Norman S (1989) Large loop excision of the transformation zone (LLETZ). A new method of management for women with cervical intraepithelial neoplasia. *Br J Obstet Gynaecol* **57**: 145

Whiteley PF, Olah KS (1990) Treatment of cervical intraepithelial neoplasia. Experience with low voltage diathermy loop. *J Obstet Gynaecol* **162**: 1272–7

Wright T, Richart R, Kjoulos J (1992) Comparison of specimens removed by CO_2 laser conization and the loop electrosurgical excision procedure. *Obstet Gynecol* **79**: 147–53

4 The polycystic ovary syndrome: pathogenesis

MC White, EI Turner

Hirsutism, oligomenorrhoea/amenorrhoea, and infertility are common clinical problems for gynaecologists and endocrinologists. When hirsutism presents with one or other of these problems, the most likely cause is the polycystic ovary syndrome (PCOS).

Although polycystic ovaries were recognised in the nineteenth century the entity of the syndrome was first brought to the attention of the medical profession in 1935 by Stein and Leventhal who described a group of seven women suffering from amenorrhoea in association with polycystic ovaries who responded to bilateral ovarian wedge resection with the return of ovulatory cycles. After further experience with this surgical technique, it was realised that not all patients benefited from the procedure and that there may be more than one cause for the condition.

Clinical and biochemical features

Patients with polycystic ovary syndrome (PCOS) usually present at some stage in their reproductive years with a history of oligomenorrhoea/amenorrhoea, hirsutism, and/or infertility, may be obese, and may have a positive family history of these symptoms and signs. Characteristic biochemical findings include an increase in circulating concentrations of free androgen, easily detectable early to midfollicular phase plasma oestradiol and elevated oestrone concentrations. Pituitary gonadotrophins are secreted in a regular pulsatile manner akin to that seen in the follicular phase of the cycle, but fail to show the cyclical changes in either absolute concentrations, pulse frequency or amplitude that are characteristic of the normal ovulatory cycle.

Ovarian morphology

Morphologically, polycystic ovaries are enlarged with a thickened tunica albuginea and contain an excess of early forming and atretic cystic follicles both beneath the surface and scattered throughout the ovary, with an increase in total stromal tissue and a relative absence of corpora albicantia. These features are consistent with a pattern of abnormal follicular development and infrequent ovulation.

The combination of the above clinical, biochemical and ovarian features represent PCOS. In order to understand how the morphological features of PCOS may develop, it is first necessary to know how normal folliculogenesis proceeds.

Normal folliculogenesis

Primordial follicles comprise oocytes that have been arrested in the first stage of meiosis, and a surrounding layer of primitive granulosa cells. Oocytes that have not been incorporated into primordial follicles during fetal life undergo degeneration. The progression of a primordial follicle to a primary and secondary follicle requires 270 days or more. Thereafter, the growth of secondary follicles into tertiary prenatal and small antral follicles takes place over 65 days. Recruitment of the cohort of follicles from which the dominant follicle will develop occurs in the luteal phase of the preceding menstrual cycle in a regularly ovulating female, ie. over a further 20 days (Gougeon, 1986).

The majority of primordial follicles never grow during the reproductive period, but those that are recruited, by an as yet unknown mechanism, demonstrate dramatic changes in structure and function. The early changes as the primordial follicle grows into a primary and then a secondary follicle do not appear to be dependent on pituitary hormones, but on local intraovarian factors.

The development of the secondary follicle is associated with the final growth of the oocyte, and the differentiation of cells around the edge of the granulosa layer into thecal cells. The secondary follicle develops an independent blood supply which is therefore capable of responding to systemic hormones including luteinizing hormone (LH) and follicle-stimulating hormone (FSH).

In the tertiary stage, an antrum forms which contains follicular fluid. This increases in size from 0.2 mm in diameter until it eventually becomes a single dominant follicle of 16–20 mm before ovulation. Throughout the reproductive years, atresia of the majority of primary, secondary and tertiary follicles takes place at a regular rate. The mechanisms controlling atresia are not clearly understood, but only the follicle that becomes dominant contains a very high concentration of oestradiol.

Folliculogenesis in polycystic ovaries

An excellent morphological review of polycystic ovarian tissue removed during wedge resection and compared with ovaries from normal women (Hughesdon, 1982) has shown that while the number of primordial follicles is similar in both groups, polycystic ovaries contain an increased number of primary, secondary and tertiary follicles. A careful review of individual findings from these data shows that while a third or so of women with polycystic ovaries have a greater number of primary and secondary follicles than normals, 80% have an increased number of early tertiary follicles. However, as the size of the follicles increases beyond 2 mm, there is a relative decline in the number of these more mature follicles.

The findings suggest two basic defects in polycystic ovaries:

1. There is either an increased recruitment of follicles or a decrease in natural atresia during early folliculogenesis up to and including the development of early tertiary follicles.
2. Atresia of tertiary follicles is accelerated compared with that in normal women, and further follicle maturation is impeded.

Atresia of secondary and tertiary follicles results in the preservation of functionally active thecal interstitial cells, which hypertrophy and maintain an active steroidogenic capacity and are responsive to pituitary LH stimulation. These cells contribute to the increased stroma of the polycystic ovary and its enhanced capacity to manufacture and secrete androgens. In addition, the same morphological study showed that there is often an increased concentration of hilar interstitial cells in women with polycystic ovaries. These hilar cells are similar to Leydig cells, appear around the time of puberty, and again secrete testosterone in response to LH. Polycystic ovaries therefore contain an increased volume of tissue capable of producing androgen which may act locally as a paracrine factor or be secreted into the systemic circulation.

The morphology of the typical polycystic ovary can thus be distinguished from that of the normal ovary using a number of parameters. The findings indicate disordered folliculogenesis. The factors that prevent orderly follicular growth have been the subject of research since PCOS was first described and will now be discussed.

Hormonal factors affecting folliculogenesis

It is not clear what causes the increase in the total number of follicles in PCOS, or what then promotes the atresia and prevents further follicular maturation. However, some inferences can be drawn from animal experiments. In hypophysectomised rats, oestrogen alone promotes preantral follicular development in the absence of endogenous gonadotrophins (Payne and Hellbaum, 1955). Androgens, when given systemically or produced locally through LH stimulation, will induce follicular atresia; administration of FSH prevents this effect (Louvet *et al*, 1975; Hillier *et al*, 1980). Thus it is possible that oestrogen alone could be responsible for increasing recruitment or preventing atresia of primary, secondary and preantral follicles in women with PCOS, while an excessive androgen concentration together with a relative insufficiency of FSH, or FSH action, could account for atresia and the failure of further follicular development.

Evidence for hormonal abnormalities in PCOS

Oestrogens

Oestradiol levels are not elevated in PCOS, but are easily detectable in concentrations similar to those found in the early midfollicular phase of the menstrual cycle. However, there is less fluctuation than in the normal cycle with neither the sharp increase that occurs at midcycle nor the fall at the end of the luteal phase. Furthermore, oestrone concentrations are generally significantly increased in PCOS (McKenna *et al*, 1985). Thus the polycystic ovary is constantly exposed to oestrogen; if this is important in recruiting or preventing atresia of primary, secondary or early tertiary follicles, it could clearly be of relevance to the pathogenesis of the condition. Other authors have proposed that continuous exposure of the pituitary to oestrone results in sensitisation to gonadotrophin-releasing hormone (GnRH) and thus increased LH release (Yen, 1980; McKenna, 1988).

Androgens

Hyperandrogenaemia is associated with the clinical and ovarian morphological features of PCOS in the majority of cases. Androgens are derived either from the adrenal gland or the ovary.

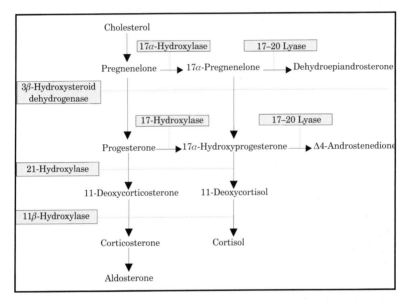

Figure 1. Adrenal steroid pathways (... denotes site of enzyme action)

The adrenal gland

The steroidogenic pathways of the adrenal gland are outlined in Figure 1. There are three main mechanisms through which adrenal androgen production may be increased:

1.   If there is a block in the synthesis of cortisol because of an enzymatic defect in the synthetic pathways. This results in a build-up of precursors which are converted to androgens through alternative pathways.

2. If there is an increase in the activity of the enzymes leading to androgen production.
3. If there is an increased requirement for cortisol which results in increased adrenocorticotrophic hormone (ACTH) stimulation of the adrenal gland (Table 1).

Table 1. Adrenal abnormalities resulting in hyperandrogenaemia

Deficiency of enzyme activity	21-hydroxylase
	3β-hydroxysteroid dehydrogenase
	11β-hydroxylase
Increased enzyme activity	17–20 lyase
Increased requirements of cortisol	Deficiency of 11β-reductase
	Enhanced 5α-reductase activity

Enzymic blocks: In specific populations, especially in the USA, late-onset congenital adrenal hyperplasia (LOCAH) associated with 21-hydroxylase, 3β-hydroxysteroid dehydrogenase or 11β-hydroxylase deficiency is a common cause of the features of PCOS, but this is not so in the UK. Nevertheless, in the UK late-onset 21-hydroxylase deficiency may be found in around 2–6% of patients with oliogomenorrhoea or hirsutism (Hague *et al*, 1989; Turner *et al*, 1992).

Increased enzyme activity: Abnormalities of adrenal androgen secretion other than those due to LOCAH can frequently be demonstrated in women with PCOS (Lucky *et al*, 1986; Turner *et al*, 1992). The findings may be due to an increase in 17–20 lyase enzyme activity, or alternatively to an increase in the volume of adrenal androgen-producing tissue (the zona reticularis of the adrenal) responsive to ACTH. A physiological increase in adrenal androgen secretion to ACTH occurs at puberty of cortisol (Genazzani *et* *al*, 1979; Schiebinger *et al*, 1981) and it has been proposed that this process may be exaggerated and prolonged in some women with PCOS.

Increased requirements for cortisol: An extremely rare cause (to date) of increased androgen production and PCOS is failure of the 11β-reductase enzyme to convert cortisone to cortisol (Phillipou and Higgins, 1985). The 11β-hydroxysteroid dehydrogenase catalyses the oxidation of the active glucocorticoid cortisol to cortisone, especially in the kidney, thus preventing cortisol activating the mineralocorticoid receptors in this organ and causing the syndrome of apparent inappropriate mineralocorticoid excess. Reversal (reduction) of this process is, however, necessary to maintain systemic cortisol levels and when this does not occur there is a decrease in negative feedback from the adrenal gland resulting in compensated hypersecretion of ACTH, and thus an increase in the activity of all the enzyme pathways leading to cortisol production.

Increased conversion of cortisol to cortisone also occurs in obese women (Mauvais-Jarvis, 1986). Thus obesity could play a role in enhancing ACTH secretion; in some women an increased metabolic clearance of cortisol due to enhanced 5α-reductase activity has been proposed as a cause of hyperandrogenaemia and PCOS (Stewart *et al*, 1990).

The ovary

Many studies have shown that the ovary is a major source of the androgens causing hyperandrogenaemia in women with polycystic ovaries. Occasional case reports have indicated a partial defect of 3β-hydroxysteroid dehydrogenase occurring in both the adrenal gland and the ovary (Axelrod *et al*, 1965; Rosenfield *et al*, 1980), but this is uncommon. There is a suggestion that enhanced activity of the 17–20-lyase enzyme occurs in the ovary, as has been proposed for the adrenal gland (Rosenfield *et al*, 1990), but whether this can explain the development of PCOS is debated, and the finding could simply be a consequence of chronic anovulation.

What is clear, however, is that the ovaries of patients with PCOS have more steroid-producing cells, as discussed earlier, and that these may be influenced by a number of exogenous factors including LH which may account directly for the hyperandrogenaemia. In addition, these secondary interstitial cells and the nests of hilar cells are closely associated with the innervation of the ovary. It is possible that direct stimulation of these cells by neurotransmitters produced locally in the ovary may also be responsible for an increase in androgen production, and for other factors that prevent the formation of a dominant follicle (Erickson et al, 1985).

Insulin and insulin-like growth factors

The relevance of hyperinsulinaemia to the development and maintenance of the polycystic ovaries is under much debate at present since hyperinsulinaemia is common in women with PCOS whether they are obese or of normal body weight (Dunaif et al, 1989). However, as with many other biochemical features of the syndrome, it is not a universal finding. Marked hyperinsulinaemia occurring in the presence of antibodies to the insulin receptor or functional defects of the insulin receptor has long been associated with the clinical and biochemical features of PCOS, these conditions being grouped together as the HAIR-AN syndrome (hyperandrogenaemia, insulin resistance, and acanthosis nigricans), but are rare (Barbieri and Ryan, 1983). In these cases it has been assumed that the hyperandrogenaemia is most likely due to an indirect effect of insulin acting through the insulin-like growth factor (IGF-1) receptor, which is known to directly enhance LH-mediated thecal cell androgen production (Cara and Rosenfield, 1988; Hernandez et al, 1988). However, in vitro, insulin can directly stimulate androgen secretion from polycystic ovaries but not from normal ovaries (Barbieri et al,

1986). Furthermore, increasing insulin levels in hyperinsulinaemic women with hyperandrogenaemia causes a direct increase in androstenedione and testosterone levels which does not occur in hyperandrogenaemic women without hyperinsulinaemia (Smith *et al*, 1987).

However, the data on the effects of insulin on androgens are not entirely consistent. In normal women, insulin may also elevate androstenedione levels acutely (Stuart *et al*, 1987). One interesting observation is that adrenal steroid production is altered in hyperinsulinaemic women who show increased androstenedione and 17α-hydroxyprogesterone responses to ACTH stimulation compared with normals (Lanzone *et al*, 1992). This could explain the possible increase in adrenal enzyme activity found in many women with PCOS.

An important consequence of hyperinsulinaemia is the direct suppression by insulin of the hepatic production of sex-hormone-binding globulin (SHBG) (Plymate *et al*, 1988). This protein, which binds testosterone, largely determines the concentration of free 'bioavailable' androgen. If excess androgen is involved in follicle atresia, this would certainly be one mechanism by which hyperinsulinaemia could be important. Likewise IGF-1-binding protein levels are inversely correlated with insulin, hyperinsulinaemia resulting in low levels of the binding protein (Suikkari *et al*, 1988; Conway *et al*, 1990). IGF-1-binding protein levels are indeed reduced in the follicular fluid of women with polycystic ovaries compared with the fluid from matched normal follicles (Holly *et al*, 1990). This could theoretically result in more bioactive IGF-1 which, as mentioned earlier, has been shown to have stimulatory effects on ovarian androgen production, and in animal models on adrenal androgens as well (Penhoat *et al*, 1989).

Suppression of hyperandrogenaemia and gonadotrophins with long-acting GnRH analogues does not alter insulin concentrations in women with PCOS (Geffner *et al*,

1986), suggesting that the hyperinsulinaemia of PCOS is independent of other hormonal changes. The presence of hyperinsulinaemia may be important for other reasons, since long-term follow-up of patients with PCOS indicates they are at greater risk of developing diabetes mellitus and ischaemic heart disease (Dahlgren *et al*, 1992).

Pituitary gonadotrophins

The pituitary hormones LH and FSH are essential for promoting the selection of the dominant follicle and for ovulation. While an intact hypothalamic GnRH pulse generator is needed to stimulate pituitary gonadotrophin release, all the changes in pulsatility, amplitude and absolute concentrations of LH and FSH that occur during the normal ovulatory cycle are dependent on the ovarian hormonal changes associated with the final stages of maturation of the dominant follicle, and the subsequent development of the corpus luteum. This can be easily demonstrated both in primates and in humans, when removal of a dominant follicle or corpus luteum at any time during the cycle is followed by a hormonal pattern of gonadotrophin secretion that reverts back to the beginning of the cycle (Nilsson *et al*, 1982; Goodman and Hodgen, 1983).

Thus the pattern of gonadotrophin secretion in PCOS could be due to a primary defect in hypothalamic-pituitary control of LH and FSH overriding the physiological gonadal feedback mechanisms, or to a major defect in folliculogenesis which prevents normal ovarian responsiveness to gonadotrophins, and thus inappropriate gonadal hormonal feedback to the hypothalamus and pituitary.

Since effective therapy for reducing free androgen concentrations can result in the resumption of normal ovulatory cycles in these cases, it is more likely that ovarian dysfunction is responsible for the pattern of pituitary hormone release. However, there are some data which implicate a primary hypothalamic-pituitary abnormality. A chronobiological disturbance has been observed in the secretion of LH in pubertal girls with PCOS, who have their daily LH surges 7–8 hours later than normal girls (Zumoff *et al*, 1983; Porcu *et al*, 1987); however, the significance of this finding is unclear. Others have suggested that the LH pulse frequency in PCOS is markedly increased compared with any other stage of the menstrual cycle (Filicori *et al*, 1989), but this is disputed (Kazer *et al*, 1987; Murdoch *et al*, 1989). What is clear, however, is that LH pulse amplitude is increased, and that the hypothalamic GnRH pulse generator is certainly functioning at a rate not less than that observed in the early follicular phase of the cycle.

Women with PCOS and anovulatory cycles have higher LH levels and lower FSH levels than those who have ovulated (Baird *et al*,1977). It has long been suggested that the persistence of oestrogen in these women (much of which is derived by aromatisation from peripheral conversion of androgens) accounts for the high LH level, but the evidence for this is speculative, especially as ovulation is associated with suppression of LH levels. The change in LH following ovulation may be caused by progesterone alone, since administration of this steroid results in a fall in LH levels, and sometimes an improvement in cyclicity (Petsos *et al*, 1986). However, once anovulation is established a high LH level may increase further any ovarian androgen production which is LH dependent, and a high level of LH may itself inhibit granulosa cell growth (Delforge *et al*, 1972).

A deficiency of FSH in women with PCOS will result in a lack of follicle maturation since this hormone is essential for promoting granulosa cell growth and differentiation and oestradiol production by the dominant follicle (Richards, 1980). However, the polycystic ovary also appears to respond less efficiently to FSH than the normal ovary (de Ziegler *et al*, 1989), and while in-vitro studies show that polycystic follicles of 5 mm contain more biologically active FSH than normal follicles of a similar size, they produce considerably less oestradiol and progesterone (Erickson *et al*, 1992). This suggests that polycystic follicles may contain inhibitors to FSH action (Lee *et al*, 1990).

Thus in women with PCOS the observed pattern of pituitary gonadotrophin secretion favours an effect of LH which will stimulate androgen production and inhibit granulosa cell growth, while ambient FSH levels are unable to promote normal oestradiol and progesterone production — exactly the milieu to promote atresia of tertiary follicles and prevent formation of a dominant follicle.

Primary abnormalities of the ovary

While we have argued that hyperandrogenaemia and persistently detectable oestrogen concentrations are the most likely factors to result in PCOS, polycystic ovaries (as demonstrated by ultrasound) are found in some women with hypogonadotrophic hypogonadism who are both hypo-oestrogenic and who do not have elevated androgens (Shoham *et al*, 1992). Furthermore, when given exogenous gonadotrophins these women responded by producing multiple follicles and had an increased tendency to hyper-stimulation. This observation would certainly favour a primary ovarian disorder in at least some cases of the syndrome.

Conclusion

There are thus many hypotheses to explain the development of the features of PCOS. There is evidence to support different mechanisms, and specific endocrine disorders have been identified, but in the majority of patients the fundamental pathology remains speculative.

Key points

- Features of polycystic ovary syndrome (PCOS) include oliogmenorrhoea, infertility, hirsutism, increased free androgen concentration and polycystic ovaries. Gonadotrophins and oestradiol continue to be secreted but there is loss of the usual cyclical changes.

- Follicular development in the ovary is morphologically normal in PCOS until the early tertiary stage ($\cong 2$ mm diameter).

- The reasons for failure of further follicular maturation are not understood. There are several hypotheses, including increased intraovarian androgen production, increased adrenal androgen production and abnormal gonadotrophin secretion.

- It is likely that more than one pathology leads to the features of PCOS. Increased adrenal androgen production is clearly associated with the features of PCOS but is present in only a minority of cases.

- Hyperinsulinaemia is common in women with PCOS but the exact role of insulin in the pathogenesis of the syndrome is debated.

References

Axelrod LR, Goldzieher JW, Ross SD (1965) Concurrent 3β-hydroxysteroid dehydrogenase deficiency in adrenal and sclerocystic ovary. *Acta Endocrinol* **48**: 392–412

Baird DT, Corker CS, Davidson DW, Hunter WM, Michie EA, Van Look PFA (1977) Pituitary–ovarian relationships in polycystic ovary syndrome. *J Clin Endocrinol Metab* **45**: 798–809

Barbieri RL, Ryan KJ (1983) Hyperandrogenism, insulin resistance and acanthosis nigricans syndrome: a common endocrinopathy with distinct pathophysiologic features. *Am J Obstet Gynecol* **147**: 90–101

Barbieri RL, Makris A, Randall RW, Daniels G, Kistner RW, Ryan KJ (1986) Insulin stimulates androgen accumulation in incubations of ovarian stroma obtained from women with hyperandrogenism. *J Clin Endocrinol Metab* **62**: 904–10

Cara JF, Rosenfield RL (1988) Insulin-like growth factor-1 and insulin potentiated LH-induced androgen synthesis by rat ovarian thecal-interstitial cells. *Endocrinol* **123**: 733–9

Conway GS, Jacobs HS, Holly JMP, Wass JAH (1990) Effects of luteinizing hormone, insulin, insulin-like growth factor 1 and insulin-like growth factor small binding protein 1 in the polycystic ovary syndrome. *Clin Endocrinol (Oxf)* **33**: 593–603

Dahlgren E, Jansen PO, Johensson S *et al* (1992) Women with polycystic ovary syndrome wedge resected in 1956 to 1965. A long-term follow-up focusing on natural history and circulating hormones. *Fertil Steril* **57**: 505–13

de Ziegler D, Steingold K, Cedars M *et al* (1989) Recovery of hormone secretion after chronic gonadotrophin-releasing hormone agonist administration in women with polycystic ovarian disease. *J Clin Endocrinol Metab* **68**: 1111–17

Delforge JP, Thomas K, Roux F, Carneiro J, Ferin J (1972) Time relationships between granulosa cell growth and luteinization and plasma luteinising hormone discharge in human. 1. A morphometric analysis. *Fertil Steril* **23**: 1–11

Dunaif A, Segal KR, Futterweit W, Dobrjansky A (1989) Profound peripheral insulin resistance independent of obesity in polycystic ovary syndrome. *Diabetes* **38**: 1165–74

Erickson GF, Magoffin DA, Dyer CA, Hofeditz CA (1985) The ovarian androgen producing cells: a review of structural functional relationships. *Endocr Rev* **6**: 371–99

Erickson GF, Magoffin DA, Garzo VG, Cheung AP, Chang RJ (1992) Granulosa cells of polycystic ovaries: are they normal or abnormal? *Hum Reprod* **7**: 293–9

Filicori M, Flamigni C, Campaniello E *et al* (1989) Evidence for a specific role of GnRH pulse frequency in the control of the human menstrual cycle. *Am J Physiol* **257**: E930–6

Geffner ME, Kaplan SA, Bersch N, Golde DW, Landaw EM, Chang JR (1986) Persistence of insulin resistance in polycystic ovarian disease after inhibition of ovarian steroid secretion. *Fertil Steril* **45**: 327–33

Genazzani AR, Pintor C, Facchinetti F, Inanudi P, Maci D, Corda D

(1979) Changes throughout puberty in adrenal secretion after ACTH. *J Steroid Biochem* **11**: 571–7

Goodman AL, Hodgen GS (1983) The ovarian triad of the primate menstrual cycle. *Recent Prog Horm Res* **39**: 1–73

Gougeon A (1986) Dynamics of follicular growth in the human: a model from preliminary results. *Hum Reprod* **1**: 81–7

Hague WM, Honour JW, Adams J, Vecsei P, Jacobs HS (1989) Steroid responses to ACTH in women with polycystic ovaries. *Clin Endocrinol (Oxf)* **30**: 355–65

Hernandez ER, Resnick CE, Svoboda ME, Van Wyk JS, Payne DW, Adashi EY (1988) Somatomedin-C/insulin- like growth factor 1 as an enhancer of androgen biosynthesis by cultured rat ovarian cells. *Endocrinolology* **122**: 1603–12

Hillier SG, Zeleznik AJ, Knazek RA, Ross GT (1980) Hormonal regulation of pre-ovulatory follicle maturation in the rat. *J Reprod Fertil* **60**: 219–29

Holly JMP, Eden JA, Alaghband-Zadeh J *et al* (1990) Insulin-like growth factor binding proteins in follicular fluid from normal dominant and cohort follicles, polycystic and multicystic ovaries. *Clin Endocrinol (Oxf)* **33**: 53–64

Hughesdon PE (1982) Morphology and morphogenesis of the Stein-Leventhal ovary and so-called 'hyperthecosis'. *Obstet Gynecol Surv* **37**: 59–77

Kazer RR, Kessel B, Yen SSC (1987) Circulating luteinizing hormone pulse frequency in women with polycystic ovary syndrome. *J Clin Endocrinol Metab* **65**: 233–6

Lanzone A, Fortini A, Fulghesu AM, Caruso A, Guido M, Mancusa S (1992) Differential androgen response to adrenocorticotropic hormone stimulation in polycystic ovarian syndrome: relationship with insulin secretion. *Fertil Steril* **58**: 296–301

Lee DW, Sheldon RM, Reichert LE (1990) Identification of low and high molecular weight follicle stimulating hormone receptor binding inhibitors in human follicular fluid. *Fertil Steril* **53**: 830–5

Louvet JP, Harman SM, Schreiber JR, Ross GT (1975) Evidence for the role of androgens in follicular maturation. *Endocrinology* **97**: 366–72

Lucky AW, Rosenfield RL, McGuire J, Rudy S, Helke J (1986) Adrenal androgen hyperresponsiveness to adrenocorticotropin in women with acne and/or hirsutism; adrenal enzyme defects and exaggerated adrenarche. *J Clin Endocrinol Metab* **62**: 840–8

Mauvais-Jarvis P (1986) Regulation of androgen receptor and 5-α-reductase in the skin of normal and hirsute women. *Clin Endocrinol Metab* **15**: 307–17

McKenna TJ (1988) Pathogenesis and treatment of polycystic ovary syndrome. *N Engl J Med* **318**: 558–62

McKenna TJ, Cunningham SK, Loughlin T (1985) The adrenal cortex and virilization. *Clin Endocrinol Metab* **14**: 997–1020

Murdoch AP, Diggle AP, White MC, Kendall-Taylor P, Dunlop W (1989) LH secretion in polycystic ovary syndrome reproductibility and pulsatile secretion. *J Endocrinol* **121**: 185–91

Nilsson L, Wikland M, Hamberger L (1982) Recruitment of an ovulatory follicle in the human following follicle-ectomy and lutectomy. *Fertil Steril* **37**: 30–4

Payne RW, Hellbaum AA (1955) The effect of estrogens on the ovary of the hypophysectomized rat. *Endocrinology* **57**: 193–9

Penhoat A, Jaillard C, Saez JM (1989) Synergistic effects of corticotrophin and insulin like growth factor 1 on corticotropin receptors and corticotropin responsiveness in bovine adrenocortical cells. *Biochem Biophys Res Commun* **165**: 355–9

Petsos P, Radcliffe WA, Anderson DC (1986) Effects of medroxyprogesterone acetate in women with polycystic ovary syndrome. *Clin Endocrinol (Oxf)* **25**: 651–60

Phillipou G, Higgins BA (1985) A new defect in the peripheral conversion of cortisone to cortisol. *J Steroid Biochem* **22**: 435–6

Plymate SR, Matej LA, Jones RE, Friedl KE (1988) Inhibition of sex hormone-binding globulin production in the human hepatoma (HEP G2) cell line by insulin and prolactin. *J Clin Endocrinol Metab* **67**: 460–4

Porcu E, Venturoli S, Magrini O *et al* (1987) Circadian variations of luteinizing hormone can have two different profiles in adolescent anovulation. *J Clin Endocrinol Metab* **65**: 488–93

Richards JS (1980) Maturation of ovarian follicles: actions and interaction of pituitary and ovarian hormones on follicular cell differentiation. *Physiol Rev* **60**: 51–89

Rosenfield RL, Rich BH, Wolfsdorf J *et al* (1980) Pubertal presentation of congenital $\Delta 5 - 3\beta$ — hydroxysteroid dehydrogenase deficiency. *J Clin Endocrinol Metab* **51**: 345–53

Rosenfield RL, Barnes RB, Cara JF, Lucky AW (1990)

Dysregulation of cytochrome P450c17α as the cause of polycystic ovary syndrome. *Fertil Steril* **53**: 785–91

Schiebinger RJ, Albertson BD, Cassorla FG *et al* (1981) The developmental changes in plasma adrenal androgens during infancy and adrenarche are associated with changing activities of adrenal microsomal 17-hydroxylase and 17, 20, desmolase. *J Clin Invest* **67**: 1177–82

Shoham Z, Conway GS, Patel A, Jacobs HS (1992) Polycystic ovaries in patients with hypogonadotrophic hypo- gonadism: similarity of ovarian responses to gonadotrophin stimulation in patients with polycystic ovarian syndrome. *Fertil Steril* **58**: 37–45

Smith S, Ravnikar VA, Barbieri RL (1987) Androgen and insulin responses to an oral glucose challenge in hyperandrogenic women. *Fertil Steril* **48**: 72–7

Stein IF, Leventhal (1935) Amenorrhoea associated with bilateral polycystic ovaries. *Am J Obstet Gynecol* **29**: 181–91

Stewart PM, Shackleton CHL, Beastall GH, Edwards CRW (1990) 5α-reductase activity in polycystic ovary syndrome. *Lancet* **355**: 431–3

Stuart CA, Prince NJ, Peters EJ, Meyer WJ (1987) Hyperinsulinemia and hyperandrogenemia: in vivo androgen responses to insulin infusion. *Obstet Gynecol* **69**: 921–5

Suikkari RM, Koivisto VA, Rutanen EM, Yki-Jarvinen H, Karonen SL, Seppala M (1988) Insulin regulates the serum levels of low molecular weight insulin-like growth factor-binding protein. *J Clin Endocrinol Metab* **66**: 266–72

Turner EL, Watson MJ, Perry LA, White MC (1992) Investigation of adrenal function in women with oliogomenorrhoea and hirsutism (clinical PCOS) from the north-east of England using an adrenal stimulation test. *Clin Endocrinol (Oxf)* **36**: 389–97

Yen SSC (1980) The polycystic ovary syndrome. *Clin Endocrinol (Oxf)* **12**: 177–207

Zumoff B, Freeman R, Coupey S, Saenger P, Markowitz M, Kresna J (1983) A chronobiological abnormality in luteinizing hormone secretion in teenage girls with the polycystic ovary syndrome. *N Engl J Med* **309**: 1206–9

5 Non-surgical treatment of cervical carcinoma

ARM Sproston

Since the discovery of radium in 1898, radiotherapy has been used in the treatment of cervical cancer, and it remains the mainstay of treatment today. Chemotherapy is in its infancy and has as yet been unable to improve long-term survival, despite encouraging response.

Carcinoma of the uterine cervix is the second commonest female cancer worldwide, with approximately 460,000 new cases each year. In the UK 4034 new cases were registered in 1991, making it the eighth commonest cancer in women, with an annual incidence of 157 per million population.

Although this article concerns non-surgical management of cervical carcinoma, it is important to emphasise that only close collaboration between oncologist, radiotherapist and gynaecologist will result in optimal treatment for the patient.

Adequate staging of the disease is the cornerstone of all treatment decisions (Table 1), for which an examination under anaesthetic is mandatory. The uterus should be assessed for size and mobility and the parametrium assessed for invasion. Rectal examination may give useful information concerning the spread of disease to the pelvic side wall and the uterosacral ligaments. Cystoscopy will determine the extent of bladder invasion in stage IV disease. A biopsy of the lesion must be taken for histological examination. An intravenous urogram may reveal ureteric obstruction. Lymphangiography, although used in North America, is not a routine investigation in the UK. Computed tomography is useful in defining the extent of bulky pelvic disease and para-aortic nodal disease, but is of little use in the assessment of patients with early stage disease. Magnetic resonance imaging may prove to be more useful in assessing local and nodal disease.

Table 1. Staging of cervical carcinoma	
Stage	
0	Intraepithelial carcinoma
I	The carcinoma is confined to the cervix
Ia	Preclinical carcinoma of the cervix, ie. those diagnosed only by microscopy
Ia1	Minimal microscopically evident stromal invasion
Ia2	Lesions detected microscopically that can be measured; the upper limit of the measurement should not show a depth of invasion of greater than 5 mm taken from the base of the epithelium, either surface or glandular, from which it originates; a second dimension, the horizontal spread, must not exceed 7 mm; larger lesions should be staged as Ib
Ib	Lesions of greater dimension than stage Ia2, whether seen clinically or not; pre-formed space involvement should not alter the staging but should be specifically recorded so as to determine whether it should affect treatment decisions in the future
II	The carcinoma extends beyond the cervix, but has not extended on to the pelvic wall; the carcinoma involves the vagina, but not as far as the lower third

IIa	No obvious parametrial involvement
IIb	Obvious parametrial involvement
III	The carcinoma has extended on to the pelvic wall, on rectal examination there is no cancer-free space between the tumour and the pelvic wall; the tumour involves the lower third of the vagina; all cases with a hydronephrosis or non-functioning kidney should be included, unless they are known to be due to another cause
IIIa	No extension on to the pelvic wall, but involvement of the lower third of the vagina
IIIb	Extension on to the pelvic wall or hydronephrosis or non-functioning kidney
IV	The carcinoma has extended beyond the true pelvis or has clinically involved the mucosa of the bladder or rectum
IVa	Spread of the growth to adjacent organs
IVb	Spread to distant organs
From FIGO (1989), reported in Shepherd (1989)	

Treatment

Most patients with stage Ia disease will be treated with surgery alone, unless the patient is unfit, in which case radiotherapy is used.

A significant number of patients with small volume stage I and IIa disease will be treated by radical hysterectomy. Some cases, however, will be treated with radiotherapy. Intracavitary therapy is usually used for early stage disease; however, intracavitary therapy alone is not curative in bulky stage Ib and II and III disease. External beam therapy is therefore used as adjunctive treatment. The decision to use adjunctive therapy with external beam irradiation depends mainly on the risk of lymph node metastasis (Table 2).

If the chances of regional disease are greater than 20%, external beam radiotherapy would be recommended. However, if the chance is less than 10%, adjunctive radiotherapy would not be appropriate. If adverse prognostic factors are present (ie. bulky tumour, lymphatic or vascular space invasion, deep penetration, poorly differentiated tumour, small cell tumour), local pelvic radiation may be considered. Unless there are problems controlling haemorrhage, external beam therapy is used initially. This causes some tumour shrinkage and may restore the anatomy of the cervical canal to a normal configuration, which allows easier insertion of the intracavitary sources. Stage IV disease is uncommon and is often treated with palliative radiotherapy, although, rarely, occasional tumours may be cured by radical radiotherapy.

Table 2. Incidence of lymph node metastasis by stage	
Stage	**Incidence**
Ia1	0%
Ia2	4.2%
Ib	18%
IIa	27%
IIb	36%
III	43%
IV	55%
From Sevin *et al* (1992)	

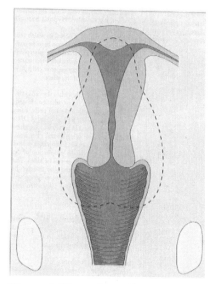

Figure 1. 'Pear-shaped' treatment area around cervix

In planning therapy, the two main factors that need to be considered are the tolerance of the tissues to radiation and the volume of the tumour. The main routes of spread of cervical cancer are laterally into the parametria and vertically into the uterus and vagina; consequently the volume of tissue to be irradiated resembles a flattened pear shape (Figure 1).

The Manchester Radium System was designed to encompass this theory and comprises a uterine applicator and vaginal ovoids (Figure 2). A point 2 cm lateral to the cervical canal and 2 cm proximal to the epithelium of the lateral vaginal fornix in the axis of the uterus is defined as point A and represents the dose to the paracervical triangle. Using the Manchester technique, for intracavitary therapy alone, point A receives 75–85 Gy (1 Gy=100 rad) in 10 days, as the uterus, cervix and vagina are relatively tolerant to radiation (Hunter, 1991). External beam therapy is used as an adjunct to intracavitary therapy and can be given in a homogeneous fashion, or graduated central shielding can be used to match the intracavitary dosimetry.

External beam therapy may be given in three ways:
1.	Parametrial X-ray therapy, which gives 50% of the prescribed dose to point A and 100% of dose given to the pelvic side wall. A total of 3250 cGy is given over 21 days

in 16 equal fractions, followed by 6000 cGy to point A in two equal intracavitary applications, over 10 days.

2. Hexagonal technique, which is designed to treat the whole pelvis and lymph nodes from the level of the top of the 5th lumbar vertebrae to the level of the lowest extent of disease in the vagina. A dose of 4000 cGy is given to the central pelvic volume, in 20 fractions over 28 days, followed by 3750 cGy as a single intracavitary dose, as soon as possible following external beam treatment.

3. Pelvic brick technique, in which a box-shaped field is applied in four directions, giving a homogeneous dose to the pelvis. Over 28 days 4000–4500 cGy is given in 20 fractions, supplemented by a single 2500 cGy intracavitary dose to point A within 2 weeks of the external beam therapy. Unfortunately, severe acute reactions are more common with this technique. However, it may be useful in patients in whom technical problems with the intracavitary sources may be anticipated.

If these fields are extended significantly beyond the true pelvis, there is an increasing morbidity, with no improvement in survival.

The response of tumours to radiotherapy depends on a number of factors.

The dose-rate effect

When the radiation dose rate is reduced from 1 Gy/min to 0.3 Gy/h there is a reduction in the cell killing resulting from a given dose, because sublethal damage repair occurs during the protracted exposure, thus decreasing the number of tumour cells killed.

The oxygen effect

The presence or absence of oxygen influences the biological effects of radiation, with the effects of radiation being greater

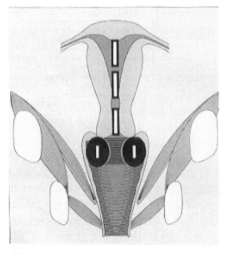

Figure 2. Positioning of intracavitary sources and vaginal ovoids

in well oxygenated tissues. To have an effect, oxygen must be present during the radiation exposure, or at least during the lifetime of the free radicals created by the radiation, and acts by the irreversible formation of organic peroxides within the DNA of the cell. Within tumours there may be areas of hypoxia and necrosis. At a distance of 150–200 μm from a capillary, the oxygen concentration is too low for viability; however, at the end of the oxygen diffusion range, there may be cells which are resistant to killing by radiation. Hypoxic fractions are typically 15–20%.

Reoxygenation may occur, in which cells that were previously hypoxic become oxygenated and are therefore more susceptible to a further dose of radiation. Fractionated radiation schedules may improve cell killing by taking advantage of this effect.

Reassortment of cells within the cell cycle

The sensitivity of a cell to radiation, depends on its position within the cell cycle, being most resistant in late S phase (time of DNA synthesis) and late G1 or G0 (resting phase when cells are out of cycle) and most sensitive in G2 and M phase. Following a dose of radiation, a significant proportion of the cells in G2 and M phase will be killed. This stimulates cells in G0 and they re-enter the cell cycle. A further dose of radiation will then be able to kill these cells when they reach G2 and M phase.

Repopulation

Treatment with radiation, or any cytotoxic agent, can trigger surviving cells in a tumour to divide faster than before. A similar phenomenon exists within normal tissues.

Intrinsic radiosensitivity

Recent work on cervical tumours (Davidson *et al*, 1990) has shown that there is a large interindividual variation in response to radiotherapy and that those tumours that are more likely to recur are more radioresistant on in-vitro testing. A similar variation has been demonstrated with in-vitro radiosensitivity testing of skin fibroblasts derived from patients treated with radiotherapy. Some fibroblast strains from patients who experienced adverse side effects from radiotherapy for breast cancer were significantly more sensitive on in-vitro testing (Burnet *et al*, 1992). These observations raise the possibility that pretreatment in-vitro testing of normal tissue radiosensitivity may identify the more radiosensitive individuals. This, in turn, may allow these patients to be treated with a reduced dose, thus decreasing the incidence of severe complications. Those patients whose normal tissues are radioresistant could receive a higher radiation dose. Suit *et al* (1989) calculated that a dose escalation of 7 or 18% could lead to an increase in the tumour control probability of 14 or 36% respectively. Increased local control and cure with unchanged or even improved normal tissue complications would result from such individualised treatment programmes.

Complications

Complications may be divided into major or minor events.

Although there are no universally accepted definitions for these terms, it is generally accepted that major complications are those that either cause prolonged morbidity or require surgical intervention. Patients receiving large volume and/or high-dose treatment are more likely to experience severe complications, but some degree of bowel and bladder dysfunction is inevitable in all patients. Pre-existing systemic diseases such as diabetes and hypertension, or a past history of pelvic infection or surgery, predispose to the development of complications. Most radiation-induced complications can be further subdivided into two groups: early and late events.

Early complications

Uterine perforation may occur during insertion of intracavitary sources. Should this not be recognised, the insertions may cause severe bowel reactions as well as signs of haemorrhage or infection. The rectum, sigmoid colon and terminal small bowel may all fall within the radiotherapy field. During the later part of the treatment cycle and the following month, this may lead to increasing frequency and irritability of the bowel, causing diarrhoea, tenesmus and occasionally intestinal obstruction. Cystitis may develop secondary to prolonged catheterisation. There will also be a degree of radiation-induced cystitis, which usually resolves within 4 weeks following treatment. All patients who are premenopausal before therapy will undergo an induced menopause, as the ovaries fall into the radiation field. Hormone replacement therapy is indicated, if there are no other contraindications, in both squamous and adenocarcinomas.

The upper vagina, and sometimes its whole length, often has an acute reaction to radiotherapy, causing adhesions at the vault and consequent vaginal stenosis. Topical oestrogen cream and the gentle use of vaginal dilators are usually sufficient treatment.

Late complications

The anterior rectal wall is a common site for problems to occur, because of its proximity to the cervix. This may present as occasional fresh bleeding with defaecation; it is usually treated with corticosteroid enemas and laxatives. Heavier bleeding may require blood transfusion and, rarely, an abdominoperineal resection. With time, increasing stenosis may cause intestinal obstruction. Patients with a redundant pelvic loop or diverticulitis are at high risk of developing these problems. Damage to the terminal ileum may present as intestinal obstruction, vague intermittent diarrhoea or possibly malabsorption syndromes with steatorrhoea.

Radiation changes within the bladder may present as painless haematuria. At diagnostic cystoscopy, telangiectases may be seen on the bladder wall, but these require no treatment unless the haemorrhage is frequent or chronic, when cautery may be used. Severe fibrosis within the bladder wall may severely reduce the bladder capacity, causing urinary frequency, which may require cystodistension, bladder augmentation or even urinary diversion.

Rare injuries include stenosis of the ureter or urethra with secondary infection, as well as vaginal telangiectasia or ulceration.

Role of chemotherapy

Chemotherapy may be used in patients with metastatic or recurrent cervical cancer. It may also have a place in the treatment of patients with early stage disease, in whom positive lymph nodes are found at laparotomy. Experimental work has also shown that chemotherapy may be used in the neoadjuvant or adjuvant setting and can also be used as a radiation potentiator. However, these approaches do not yet have an established role in routine practice. In several trials, single agent chemotherapy, with a variety of agents, has shown response rates in the range of 10–25%; several alkylating agents, doxorubicin, fluorouracil, hexamethylmelamine and methotrexate are among the most active. More recently, cisplatin has shown response rates of 20–30%.

Non-randomised trials using combination chemotherapy, including cisplatin, have shown an improved response rate of approximately 40%. However, despite the apparent increase in the response rate, the progression-free interval and survival remain disappointing. Nevertheless, occasional patients, especially those with only pulmonary metastases, show a long disease-free survival, or may even be cured (Burnet and Blake, 1989).

Neoadjuvant chemotherapy

Neoadjuvant chemotherapy (NACT) (given before radiotherapeutic or surgical intervention) may prove useful in debulking tumour and in eradicating subclinical metastases. Early trials, however, have shown no improvement in survival with NACT and radiotherapy combined. This may be due to an accelerated regrowth of surviving clones following chemotherapy, or to the development of cross-resistance to certain chemotherapeutic agents and radiotherapy. The results of NACT before surgery seem to be more encouraging. The incidence of positive pelvic lymph nodes in stage Ib–IIa disease following NACT varied from 6 to 23%. This compares favourably with earlier reports of between 40 and 80% lymph node involvement in patients with bulky stage Ib–IIa who did not receive NACT.

Concurrent chemoradiation

Small pilot studies have shown that radiotherapy, combined with an infusion of fluorouracil, cisplatin or cisplatin combinations or hydroxyurea may improve disease-free interval and survival. Further, larger, randomised trials are required to confirm these observations.

Adjuvant chemotherapy

Adjuvant therapy may improve the prognosis in those patients who, although having early stage disease, are at increased risk of relapse following primary therapy, ie. those patients with involved para-aortic and/or pelvic lymph nodes, lymphatic or vascular invasion in the cervix, tumour size >4 cm diameter, parametrial invasion and evidence of locally metastatic disease. These patients have traditionally been treated with post-operative external beam radiotherapy. Adjuvant chemotherapy may have a useful role in the treatment of these patients, as they may be regarded as having systemic disease.

Key points

- Accurate staging is vital for optimal treatment.
- The decision to use external beam irradiation in early stage disease depends on the risk of lymph node metastasis.
- Radiotherapy is aimed at delivering a dose of 75–85 Gy to the paracervical triangle.
- Radiation-induced complications may occur early, eg. diarrhoea and cystitis, or late, eg. bladder fibrosis and bowel stenosis.
- Pre-existing systemic disease, such as diabetes and hypertension, may predispose to the development of complications with radiotherapy.
- Chemotherapy, despite some encouraging reported response rates, has, as yet, been unable to improve long-term survival.
- Following radiotherapy for both squamous cell carcinomas and adenocarcinomas in premenopausal patients, hormone replacement therapy is indicated, provided that there are no other contraindications.

References

Burnet NG, Blake PR (1989) Sustained complete remission of stage IVB carcinoma of the cervix with cisplatinum, methotrexate and bleomycin chemotherapy. *Br J Radiol* **62**: 661–3

Burnet NG, Nyman J, Turesson I, Wurm R, Yarnold JR, Peacock JH (1992) Prediction of normal tissue tolerance to radiotherapy from in vitro cellular radiation sensitivity. *Lancet* **339**: 1570–1

Davidson SE, West CML, Roberts SA, Hendry JH, Hunter RD (1990) Radiosensitivity testing of primary cervical carcinoma: evaluation of intra- and inter-tumour heterogeneity. *Radiother Oncol* **18**: 349–56

Hunter RD (1991) Female genital tract. In: Pointon RCS ed. *Radiotherapy of Malignant Disease.* 2nd edn. Springer Verlag, London: 279–308

Shepherd JH (1989) Revised FIGO staging for gynaecological cancer. *Br J Obstet Gynaecol* **96**: 889–92

Sevin B-U, Nadii M, Averette HE, Hilsenbeck S, Smith D, Lampe B (1992) Microinvasive carcinoma of the cervix. *Cancer* **70**: 2121–8

Suit HD, Baumann M, Skates S, Convery K (1989) Clinical interest in determination of cellular radiation sensitivity. *Int J Radiat Biol* **56**: 725–37

Further reading

Hall EJ (1994) *Radiobiology for the Radiologist.* 4th edn. JB Lippincott, Philadelphia

6 Primary surgical management of cervical cancer

R Kingston

Early-stage cervical cancer cancer can be readily cured by surgery, with acceptably low morbidity. Successful treatment depends on appropriate surgical training, tight organisation, thorough selection of patients, selection of the right operation and close liaison with the pathologist and radiotherapist.

Surgical intervention may be apposite at several points in the management of invasive cervical cancer: these may be broadly summarised as preventative, primary curative, salvage or palliative. This article will concentrate on primary curative surgery (Table 1).

Primary management depends on a variety of factors, including physical fitness, coincidental medical problems, clinical staging and histopathological data. Three basic questions have to be answered at the outset:

1. Is radical treatment necessary or will local treatment suffice?
2. If radical treatment is required, is surgery or radiotherapy better?
3. How radical should radical hysterectomy be?

Table 1. Surgical options for cervical cancer		
Primary	Simple	Loop excision
		Cone biopsy
		Hysterectomy
	Radical	hysterectomy

Adjunctive	Simple extrafascial hysterectomy
	Radical hysterectomy
Salvage for recurrence	Radical hysterectomy
	Exenterative procedures
Palliative, eg. diversionary procedures for fistula	

Is radical treatment necessary or will local treatment suffice?

The first question arises in cases of microinvasive or occult invasive disease diagnosed by excisional biopsy of the transformation zone, eg. knife cone or loop excision. Histopathological staging data are critical factors in determining whether the procedure is sufficient to cure. If further surgery is required, there is rarely any logic in recommending simple hysterectomy, although this operation has been widely advised in this situation in the past. When cervical cancer spreads it will usually do so into the parametrial and regional nodes, and the planned operation must take account of this. In most cases the selection of operation of choice therefore passes directly from cone biopsy to some form of radical hysterectomy, and close liaison between gynaecologist and histopathologist is essential in ensuring that the patient is appropriately treated.

If radical treatment is required, is surgery or radiotherapy better?

Delgado (1978) has reviewed this question, which has been subjected to intense and often futile debate. No difference has been observed between the two forms of treatment in the survival rates for disease of equivalent clinical stage (Hopkins and Morley, 1991). The choice therefore depends on the risks and morbidity of the treatments (Shepherd, 1990), or on logistic factors, eg. the ease of access to treatment. Surgery is usually advised for young patients who are more likely to be fit for radical procedures, who will benefit from conservation of ovarian function, and who stand to lose most if there are intractable complications of radiotherapy (Peel *et al*, 1991). The most important criteria for treatment selection are the clinical stage and the volume of the primary tumour (Table 2). The latter, although not specified in the FIGO staging protocol (Shepherd, 1989), is important since bulky tumours, whether confined to the cervix or not, are more likely to be associated with extensive node metastases. These may therefore be more suitable for radiotherapy or combined modality treatment with radiotherapy and chemotherapy. Tumour volume can be conveniently approximated at the time of clinical staging by assessing the diameter of the primary tumour. Bulky tumours can be arbitrarily defined as those >4 cm in diameter. The 4 cm rule has been recently incorporated into the latest FIGO definition of cervical cancer staging, see *BJOG,* May 1996, **103**: 405.

Table 2. Indications for primary surgery illustrated by the Liverpool protocol	
Type of cancer	**Stage**
Microinvasive carcinoma	1ai. Early stromal invasion
	1aii. Microcarcinoma
Overt carcinoma in premenopausal women	1b. Invasive cancer <4 cm diameter confined to cervix
	2a. Invasive cancer <4 cm diameter extending to vaginal fornices

How radical should radical hysterectomy be?

This question implies that the radicality of the operation can be tailored to the individual circumstances of the patient (DiSaia and Creasman, 1984). The operation itself can be regarded as a modular system of successive but essentially separate procedures performed under the same anaesthetic (Table 3).

Table 3. Modular approach to extended hysterectomy	
Module	**Treatment**
Trial dissection	Surgical restaging
Ovaries	Conserve
	Remove
	Transpose outside pelvis
Nodes	Conserve
	Sampling only
	Pelvic lymphadenectomy
	Pelvic and para-aortic lymphadenectomy
Parametrium	Conserve
	Remove medial third
	Remove medial two thirds
	Remove all to side wall
Vaginal cuff	Up to 3 cm beyond palpable cervix

The detailed technique of radical hysterectomy is beyond the scope of this article, and the reader is referred to the descriptive accounts by Averette *et al* (1984) and Monaghan (1986). In summary, most surgeons in the UK and USA follow a technique based on that of Meigs (1951), which is different from Wertheim's original operation. Piver *et al* (1974) have devised a system for grading the radicality of the operation. In Liverpool, the technique follows that of Averette *et al* with minor modifications.

The operation begins with a trial dissection, which is in effect a surgical restaging to confirm operability. This is designed so that, if the disease proves to be inoperable after all, the abdomen can be closed without compromise to any subsequent radiotherapy. If the 4 cm diameter rule is adhered to in patient selection, this eventuality should be rare. At this point the operation proceeds normally, with the surgeon clear in his/her mind regarding the management of the remaining modules of the operation: namely, the fate of the ovaries, the extent of the lymphadenectomy, the amount of ureteric mobilisation and the extent of the parametrial and vaginal cuffs.

Squamous tumours *vs* adenocarcinomas

There has been debate as to whether adenocarcinomas should be managed differently from squamous tumours. Recent reviews have concluded that the management should generally be the same, stage for stage (Ireland *et al*, 1984; Luesley, 1989). There remain, however, two particularly contentious areas of debate:

1. Microinvasion is a dubious concept in cervical adenocarcinoma because of uncertainty regarding its histological characteristics. It is probably safer to manage very early invasive disease more aggressively than its squamous counterpart. The significance of the staging criteria for the clinical management are considered in more detail below.

2. Conservation of the ovaries is more controversial since ovarian metastases in early-stage adenocarcinoma although still uncommon, are more frequent than the negligible incidence associated with squamous tumours (Toki *et al*, 1991). On balance, ovarian conservation is still reasonable, especially in very young patients (Owens *et al*, 1989). However, clinical follow-up may need to be supplemented by periodic ultrasound to

check for ovarian enlargement, and oophorectomy and postoperative hormone replacement therapy considered in patients over 40 years.

Organisational considerations

In Liverpool, the general approach to treatment outlined above has been formalised since 1990 into a general protocol. This covers all patients with cervical cancer referred to the oncology clinic of the Liverpool Women's Hospital, which is jointly supervised by a gynaecological oncologist and a radiotherapist with a specialist interest in gynaecological brachytherapy. All Liverpool gynaecologists, as well as many from the Mersey region and North Wales, refer centrally to this clinic, as do other regional radiotherapists and oncologists.

The importance of a comprehensive clincical treatment protocol, strictly adhered to and agreed in advance with both histopathologist and radiotherapist, cannot be overemphasised. Such a protocol is conveniently formulated, monitored and managed via a centralised multidisciplinary consultation clinic.

In recent years there has been an increasing perception of the need for greater subspecialisation in gynaecological cancer treatment (Royal College of Obstetricians and Gynaecologists Working Party, 1982). By attracting tertiary referrals within individual hospitals or at regional level, gynaecological surgeons with special interests in oncology acquire concentrated experience of gynaecological cancer surgery unobtainable in the course of normal referral practice. This enhanced expertise pays dividends in the selection of the most appropriate treatment, the maintenance of specialist technical skills, the deployment of those skills to achieve optimal operability rates, and not least the prevention, early identification and correct management of complications.

Furthermore, the concentration of large numbers of

patients with similar conditions following standardised clinical protocols creates ideal circumstances for post-graduate training, and also for easily organised clinical audit and research. The fundamental prerequisite for safe and effective gynaecological cancer surgery is therefore organisational. Centralisation of referrals in this way is particularly vital for procedures which are extensive, relatively high risk, and infrequently indicated, eg. radical hysterectomy, and gynaecologists who persist with the occasional performance of such operations should consider carefully whether their policy is in the best interest of their patients (Bisset *et al*, 1994).

Treatment protocol and selection criteria for surgery

Current FIGO clinical staging (Shepherd, 1989) is adhered to, with examination under anaesthetic, curettage and biopsies, cystoscopy, full blood count, urea, electrolytes and creatinine levels assessed, liver function tests and chest X-ray performed. Pelvic imaging is also required: intravenous urography in cases of tumour confidentiality thought to be confined to the cervix, abdominopelvic computed tomography or magnetic resonance imaging where parametrial involvement is suspected. The Liverpool protocol uses this staging procedure as an indication for primary surgery (Table 2).

Stage 1a. Microinvasive carcinoma

Squamous cancers only. Attempts to put adenocarcinomas into this group should be regarded with grave suspicion.

Stage 1ai. Early stromal invasion

This condition is normally diagnosed by cone biopsy and is likely to constitute effective treatment, given complete excision. Patient should have initial follow-up with 4-monthly smears for 2 years, including a colposcopic examination. Patients with cone margins involved by cervical intraepithelial neoplasia or who have completed their families or who are unusually anxious about retaining their uterus in spite of counselling may be offered total hysterectomy. There is no indication for radical hysterectomy or radiotherapy.

Stage 1aii. Microcarcinoma

This group represents the watershed between conservative and radical treatment. As follow-up data on this sub-stage accumulate, it may be possible in future to adopt a more conservative approach. However, for the present the treatment of choice is Rutledge-Meigs type 2 modified radical hysterectomy (ureters mobilised laterally taking care to conserve mesoureters, but not radically dissected, to allow a cuff of one third of parametrium) and pelvic node dissection up to the level of the iliac bifurcation. There is no indication for routine oophorectomy.

Stage 1b/2a. Non-bulky tumours (<4 cm diameter)

These are individualised on the basis of age and fitness, as discussed above. Generally, premenopausal patients will be recommended surgery and post-menopausal patients will be recommended radiotherapy.

Surgery

Rutledge-Meigs type 3 radical hysterectomy (ureters completely dissected from the cardinal ligaments, to allow excision of a minimum of two thirds lateral parametrium), with pelvic **and** para-aortic node dissection up to the origin of the inferior mesenteric artery. Suspicious para-aortic nodes are sent for frozen section and the operation abandoned in favour of radiotherapy if positive for malignancy. There is no indication for routine oophorectomy; the ovaries are managed on their own merits according to the criteria outlined above. When the ovaries are conserved, consideration should be given to transposition of one ovary (usually the right) on its vascular pedicle out of the pelvis into the paracolic gutter, the vessels being laid behind the caecum. This is performed to reduce the risk of radiation menopause in those patients requiring postoperative radiotherapy.

Radiotherapy as an adjunct to radical hysterectomy

Preoperative radiotherapy is now widely regarded as outmoded and unnecessary.

The status of postoperative radiotherapy also remains controversial, as the practice originally evolved uncritically and is not based on the results of clinical trials. The evidence that exists indicates that postoperative radiotherapy reduces the risk of pelvic recurrence but has little effect on eventual prognosis (Morrow, 1980). Conversely, surgery alone is capable of curing some node-positive patients. Furthermore, the incidence of serious complications is higher when radical radiotherapy follows radical surgery (Rutledge *et al*, 1976).

A tightly observed selection protocol and the 4 cm rule help to reduce to a minimum those cases in which post-operative radiotherapy is deemed advisable.

The chief risk factors for postoperative recurrence are involved surgical margins and node positivity. Other factors, eg. histological characteristics, rarely need to be taken into account following a comprehensive lymphadenectomy.

Involved margins should be an exceptionally rare occurrence in a well-conducted series of operations.

Node positivity, consisting of micrometastases only in one or two nodes, receives only expectant management in our protocol, with postoperative radiotherapy reserved for more extensive pelvic node involvement.

Key points

- Early-stage cervical cancer can be very successfully treated by surgery.

- The selection of the right operation for the right patient requires careful planning and multidisciplinary liaison.

- Radical hysterectomy and lymphadenectomy, with conservation of the ovaries, is the surgical management of choice in most cases.

- The extent of the surgery can be judged according to individual patient characteristics.

- Patients whose histology results indicate a high risk of pelvic recurrence may be offered postoperative therapy.

References

Averette HE, Ford JH, Girtanner RE, Sevin BU (1984) Radical hysterectomy. In: Nyhus L, Baker R, eds. *Mastery of Surgery*. Little Brown and Co, Toronto: 1183–93

Bisset D, Lamont DW, Nwabineli NJ, Brodie MM, Symonds RP (1994) Treatment of stage 1 carcinoma cervix in the west of Scotland 1980–1987. *Br J Obstet Gynaecol* **101**: 615–20

Delgado G (1978) Stage 1b squamous cancer of the cervix: the choice of treatment. *Obstet Gynecol Survey* **33**: 174–83

DiSaia PJ, Creasman WT, eds (1984) Invasive cervical cancer: surgical management. *Clincial Gynecologic Oncology*. 2nd edn. CV Mosby Co, St Louis: 76–85

Hopkins MP, Morley GW (1991) Radical hysterectomy *vs* radiation therapy for stage 1b squamous cell carcinoma cervix. *Cancer* **68**: 272–7

Ireland D, Hardiman P, Monaghan JM (1984) Adenocarcinoma of the uterine cervix: a study of 73 cases. *Obstet Gynecol* **65**: 82–5

Luesley D (1989) Cervical adenocarcinoma. In: Studd J, ed. *Progress in Obstetrics and Gynaecology*. Vol 7. Churchill Livingstone, Edinburgh: 369–88

Meigs JV (1951) Radical hysterectomy with bilateral pelvic node dissection. *Am J Obstet Gynecol* **62**: 854–66

Monaghan JM, ed (1986) Radical hysterectomy and pelvic node dissection. *Bonney's Gynaecological Surgery.* 9th edn. Bailliere Tindall, London: 95–107

Morrow CP (1980) Panel report: is pelvic radiation beneficial in the postoperative management of stage 1b squamous cell carcinoma cervix? *Gynecol Oncol* **10**: 105–10

Owens S, Roberts WS, Fiorica JV, Hoffman MS, Lapolla JP, Cavanagh D (1989) Ovarian management at the time of radical hysterectomy for cancer of the cervix. *Gynecol Oncol* **35**: 349–51

Peel KR, Khoury GG, Joslin CAF *et al* (1991) Cancer of the cervix in women under 40 years of age. *Br J Obstet Gynaecol* **98**: 993–1000

Piver MS, Rutledge F, Smith JP (1974) Five classes of extended hysterectomy for women with cervical cancer. *Obstet Gynecol* **44**: 265–72

Royal College of Obstetricians and Gynaecologists Working Party (1982) *Further Specialisation Within Obstetrics and Gynaecology.* Royal College of Obstetricians and Gynaecologists, London

Rutledge FN, Wharton JT, Fletcher GH (1976) Clinical studies with adjunctive surgery and irradiation therapy in the treatment of carcinoma of the cervix. *Cancer* **38**: 596–602

Shepherd JH (1989) Revised FIGO staging for gynaecological cancer. *Br J Obstet Gynaecol* **97**: 889–92

Shepherd JH (1990) Cervical cancer: the surgical management of early stage disease. In: Shepherd JH, Monaghan JM, eds. *Clinical Gynaecological Oncology.* 2nd edn. Blackwell Scientific Publications, Oxford: 64–7

Toki N, Tsukamoto N, Kaku T *et al* (1991) Microscopic ovarian metastasis of cervical cancer. *Gynecol Oncol* **41**: 46–51

7 Management of post-term pregnancy: to induce or not?

Z Alfirevic, SA Walkinshaw

Perinatal mortality is increased in pregnancies over 42 weeks, but can be reduced by the induction of labour. However, clinicians must consult with the patient as to whether she would rather experience spontaneous onset of labour or accept this increased risk. This chapter weighs up the important considerations in this difficult area.

The definition of post-term pregnancy endorsed by the World Health Organisation (1977) and the International Federation of Gynaecology and Obstetrics (FIGO) (1984) is 42 completed weeks or more (≥ 294 days). Post-term pregnancy and other terms used synonymously such as prolonged pregnancy, post-dates or after-term pregnancy are, therefore, statements about the chronological duration of pregnancy. They do not infer pathological condition and should not be confused with the term 'post-maturity' which refers to features seen occasionally in infants born after prolonged gestation (loss of subcutaneous fat, dry and cracked skin, meconium staining of the skin, etc) (Clifford, 1954). The reported incidence of post-term pregnancy ranges from 4 to 14%, with an average of about 10% (Bakketig and Bergsjo, 1989). Post-term pregnancy appears to be more common in primigravidae and women with previous post-term births.

Evidence gathered over the last 60 years shows that perinatal mortality is higher if pregnancy goes beyond 42 weeks (Bakketig and Bergsjo, 1989; Crowley, 1989). However, the magnitude of this increase remains controversial. Large observational data on term and post-term births from

Scandinavia suggest that the number of perinatal deaths is lowest at 40 weeks' gestation (0.23%), with only a slight increase to 0.30% at 42 weeks and 0.40% at 43 weeks (Bakketig and Bergsjo, 1989). Several case series have failed to confirm this unfavourable trend but these have been smaller studies and merely highlight the rarity of perinatal deaths and the need for large numbers to show a statistically significant difference (Crowley, 1989).

The increase in perinatal deaths in post-term pregnancy is caused by a range of factors, including congenital malformations, perinatal infections and anoxic conditions such as placental abruption, Rhesus disease and intrauterine growth retardation (Lucas *et al*, 1965; Naeye, 1978). Failure to take into account that around one quarter of post-term deaths could be ascribed to congenital malformations (Naeye, 1978) results in an overestimation of the risk of potentially avoidable perinatal death after 42 weeks relative to that at term. On the other hand, the overall risk of post-term pregnancy may be significantly underestimated because most high-risk pregnancies (twins, pre-eclampsia, Rhesus disease, growth retardation) will be electively delivered before 42 weeks. Unfortunately, large, case-controlled, matched comparisons of entirely normal term and post-term pregnancies have not been published.

Faced with this epidemiological data, parents and clinicians are left with two options. One is to interrupt pregnancy before it goes post-term, hoping that induction of labour will prevent development of the risk factors that increase perinatal mortality. The alternative is expectant management with adequate fetal monitoring to ensure that intervention is restricted to pregnancies that will benefit from it. Although the choice between the two policies appears to be simple, it affects around 80 000 women in the UK each year and has serious implications, including parent satisfaction and cost-effectiveness.

There follows a review of currently available information

about these two policies with an emphasis on the evidence from randomised controlled trials (RCTs) gathered by the Cochrane Collaboration (Enkin *et al*, 1993).

To induce?

The data from RCTs favour a policy of inducing labour after 41 weeks' gestation (Crowley, 1993a). Meta-analysis of 13 RCTs shows a statistically significant reduction in perinatal mortality for normally formed babies and a decrease in the number of caesarean sections following 'active' management. The policy of routine induction appears to be safe and causes no increase in maternal uptake of analgesia or rates of operative vaginal delivery, meconium aspiration syndrome or neonatal seizures.

The only identified adverse effects of such active management is an increase in neonatal jaundice (Figure 1). However, the generalisability of these results has been questioned (Keirse, 1993a) because more than 50% of a pooled data comes from the recent large Canadian trial with 3407 participants (Hannah *et al*, 1992). In this trial, the caesarean section rate was 20.6% and prostaglandin E_2 (PGE_2) was not available for the group assigned to fetal surveillance because it was felt that most of the fetuses in this group would be compromised. Therefore, the overall reduction in the caesarean section rate from 21.6% to 19.5% shown in the meta-analysis by Crowley (1993a), although statistically significant, may not be relevant for obstetric units with caesarean section rates around 10% and more liberal use of PGE_2. It is possible that routine induction of labour in such units may actually have the opposite effect, causing a greater need for obstetric interventions, with all the subsequent consequences.

The observed reduction in perinatal mortality is a much more worrying finding for women and clinicians who prefer conservative management. Perinatal mortality is only

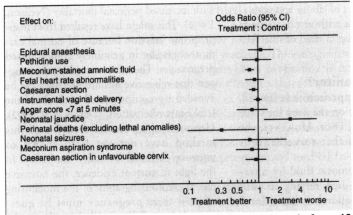

Figure 1. Graph of odds ratios and confidence intervals from 13 trials showing the effects of elective induction of labour after 41 weeks' gestation on various perinatal outcomes. The result is not significant if the confidence interval overlaps an odds ratio of 1.0. From Crowley (1993b)

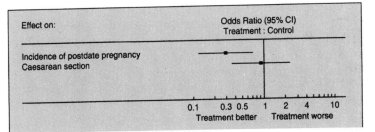

Figure 2. Effect of prolonged breast stimulation on the incidence of post-term pregnancies and caesarean sections from one trial. The result is not significant if the confidence interval overlaps an odds ratio of 1.0. From Crowley (1993b)

around 2 per 1000 in pregnancies after 41 weeks (Grubb *et al*, 1992; Crowley, 1993a) but it may drop to 0.3 per 1000 with routine induction. Although statistically significant, this effect may well be due to chance, bearing in mind that the analysed RCTs did not use perinatal mortality as their primary endpoint. Even if the reduction in perinatal mortality following active management is real, many women require intervention in order to achieve it (500 inductions to prevent one perinatal death). Women's views on the acceptability of an increased intervention rate for gains of this nature have yet to be obtained.

If induction of labour is favoured it would be interesting to know whether this can be achieved without surgical or pharmacological intervention. Evidence from one small trial with 200 randomised women suggests that nipple stimulation for 3 hours per day from 39 weeks until delivery decreases the incidence of post-term pregnancy (Figure 2) (Elliot and Flaherty, 1984). Another potentially useful procedure is sweeping or stripping of the membranes during vaginal examination at term. The chances of spontaneous onset of labour within 3 days of vaginal examination are doubled if the membranes are swept (Allot and Palmer, 1993). Unfortunately, trials have been too small to discover the effect of sweeping of the membranes on the mode of delivery and perinatal outcome (Grant, 1993). There is currently no evidence that sexual intercourse can shorten the duration of pregnancy, despite the high prostaglandin content of seminal plasma (Keirse, 1993b).

The state of the cervix commonly influences the decision about induction of labour. It is commonly believed that labour is best induced if the cervix is favourable because an easy and uncomplicated induction may be anticipated. On the other hand, if the cervix is unfavourable the pregnancy is monitored while waiting for spontaneous ripening of the cervix. It is possible that such a policy is exactly opposite to what is best for women. If there is a causal link between delayed onset of labour and perinatal mortality, women with unripe cervixes may be the very group in need of intervention.

To monitor?

If a conservative approach is favoured, most clinicians agree on the need for some sort of fetal surveillance. However, the type and timing of that surveillance is unclear.

Assessment of amniotic fluid by ultrasound is commonly used, relying on early evidence of an association between reduced amniotic fluid volume and perinatal morbidity (Crowley *et al*, 1984). The definition of reduced amniotic fluid volume on ultrasound examination varies and the decision on whether to use subjective assessment, maximum pool depth or amniotic fluid index is arbitrary (Figure 3). Only recently have attempts been made to determine the most efficacious cut-off points using receiver-operator curves (ROCs) (Chauhan *et al*, 1994). There are no reported RCTs from which to make a reliable choice of the most appropriate method of amniotic fluid volume assessment for a post-term monitoring protocol.

Despite the widespread use of either standard or computerised cardiotocography, the four published RCTs of antepartum cardiotocography provide no support for the use of this technique in high-risk pregnancies; indeed, its use

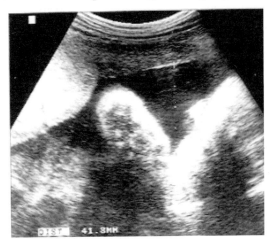

Figure 3.
Ultrasound scan showing a normal pool of amniotic fluid (42 mm) in a post-term pregnancy

appears to be associated with increased perinatal mortality (Neilson, 1993a). This might have resulted from inappropriate inaction because of normal cardiotocography in genuinely compromised pregnancies. There is some evidence to suggest that subjective misinterpretation can be avoided by computerised analysis of the fetal heart rate pattern (Dawes *et al*, 1992). However, the potential benefits of this method have not yet been shown to improve perinatal mortality/morbidity. In the light of current evidence, the extensive use of cardiotocography in the monitoring of post-term pregnancy must be questioned. Its validity is likely to lie in the assessment of immediate fetal health following events such as sudden reduction of fetal movements or antepartum haemorrhage and not in the assessment of fetal/placental 'reserve'.

More sophisticated biophysical monitoring, comprising cardiotocography and ultrasound evaluation of amniotic fluid volume and fetal breathing, tone and gross body movements (biophysical profile), has been suggested for a post-term fetal surveillance (Johnson *et al*, 1986) but observational data suggest that a combination of cardiotocography and amniotic fluid assessment performs just as well (Walkinshaw, 1993). Our recent RCT comparing the biophysical profile with a combination of cardiotocography and maximum pool depth failed to show any advantage of the use of the more complex fetal surveillance protocol (Alfirevic and Walkinshaw, 1994).

Doppler ultrasound reduces perinatal mortality in high-risk pregnancies, but stratified meta-analysis for post-term pregnancies is, at present, not possible because of the small numbers of randomised pregnancies (Neilson, 1993b). The conclusions from observational data range from clear benefit of Doppler ultrasound in the assessment of the post-term pregnancy to no benefit (Pearce and McParland, 1991; Stokes and Newnham, 1991). All of these uncertainties were discussed by the Royal College of Obstetricians and Gynaecologists Medical Audit Unit (1993) which was unable to offer guidelines on surveillance methods for pregnancy after 42 weeks because the medical evidence was insufficient. Although the current evidence suggests that simple monitoring protocols are as safe as complex ones, there is an obvious need for large RCTs to determine the most effective monitoring methods.

Third option

Parents' views and their satisfaction have been notoriously under-researched in the field of perinatal medicine. The management of term and post-term pregnancy is no exception. Parents have to choose between marginal benefit in the perinatal death rate following induction and their wish to experience spontaneous onset of labour. The choice is not an easy one and may be influenced by numerous social and medical factors.

Women vary greatly in their feelings about obstetric intervention and these feelings may change as post-term pregnancy continues. Blanket policies of induction or monitoring fail to take these factors into account and therefore seem increasingly obsolete. The public demand for a change in obstetric care cannot be ignored. Easy access to all relevant information and competent, compassionate counselling would be a good start in meeting parents' needs.

Key points

- Perinatal mortality is increased in post-term pregnancies.
- Evidence from randomised trials suggests that routine induction of labour after 41 weeks decreases perinatal mortality.
- Some parents and clinicians favour a conservative approach because up to 500 inductions may be

required to prevent one perinatal death.

- There is no consensus as to what constitutes an optimal fetal monitoring protocol in post-term pregnancy.

- The patient's choice lies between marginal reduction in perinatal deaths following induction of labour and her wish to experience spontaneous onset of labour.

- Easy access to all relevant information and compassionate counselling are necessary in order to meet parents' needs and allow them to make an informed choice.

References

Alfirevic Z, Walkinshaw SA (1995) A randomized controlled trial of simple vs complex antenatal fetal monitoring after 42 weeks gestation. *Br J Obstet Gynaecol* **102** (8):638–643

Allot HA, Palmer CR (1993) Sweeping the membranes: a valid procedure in stimulating the onset of labour? *Br J Obstet Gynaecol* **100**: 898–903

Bakketig LS, Bergsjo P (1989) Post-term pregnancy: magnitude of the problem. In: Chalmers I, Enkin M, Keirse MJNC, eds. *Effective Care in Pregnancy and Childbirth. Vol 1.* Oxford University Press, Oxford: 765–75

Chauhan SP, Cowan BD, Magann EF *et al* (1994) Intrapartum amniotic fluid index and adverse outcome: experience with 1000 parturients. *Am J Obstet Gynecol* **170**: 393

Clifford SH (1954) Postmaturity — with placental dys function. Clinical syndrome and pathological findings. *J Pediatr* **44**: 1–33

Crowley P (1989) Post-term pregnancy: induction or surveillance? In: Chalmers I, Enkin M, Keirse MJNC, eds. *Effective Care in Pregnancy and Childbirth. Vol 1.* Oxford University Press, Oxford: 776–91

Crowley P (1993a) Elective induction of labour at 41+ weeks gestation. In: Enkin MW, Keirse MJNC, Renfrew MJ, Neilson JP, eds. *Cochrane Database of Systematic Reviews.* Update Software, Oxford : review no 4144

Crowley P (1993b) Breast stimulation for the management of

post-term pregnancy. In: Enkin MW, Keirse MJNC, Renfrew MJ, Neilson JP, eds. *Cochrane Database of Systematic Reviews*. Disk Issue 2. Update Software, Oxford: review no 6860

Crowley P, O'Herlihy C, Boylan P (1984) The value of ultrasound measurement of amniotic fluid volume in the management of prolonged pregnancies. *Br J Obstet Gynaecol* **91**: 444–8

Dawes GS, Lobb M, Moulden M, Redman CWG, Wheeler T (1992) Antenatal cardiotocogram quality and interpretation using computers. *Br J Obstet Gynaecol* **99**: 791–7

Elliot JP, Flaherty JF (1984) The use of breast stimulation to prevent postdate pregnancy. *Am J Obstet Gynecol* **149**: 628–32

Enkin MW, Keirse MJNC, Renfrew MJ, Neilson JP eds (1993) *Cochrane Database of Systematic Review — Pregnancy and Childbirth Module*. Disk Issue 2. Update Software, Oxford

FIGO (1984) Report of the FIGO subcommittee on perinatal epidemiology and health statistics following a workshop in Cairo, November 11–18, 1984, on the methodology of measurement and recording of infant growth in the perinatal period. FIGO, London: 54

Grant JM (1993) Sweeping of the membranes in prolonged pregnancy. *Br J Obstet Gynaecol* **100**: 887–9

Grubb DK, Rabello YS, Paul RH (1992) Post-term pregnancy: fetal death rate with antepartum surveillance. *Obstet Gynecol* **79**: 1024–6

Hannah ME, Hannah WJ, Hellmann J, Hewson S, Milner R, Willan A (1992) Induction of labour as compared with serial antenatal monitoring in post-term pregnancy. *N Engl J Med* **326**: 1587–92

Johnson JM, Harman CR, Lange IR, Manning FA (1986) Biophysical profile scoring in the management of post-term pregnancy: an analysis of 307 patients. *Am J Obstet Gynecol* **154**: 269–73

Keirse MJNC (1993a) Post-term pregnancy: new lessons from an unresolved debate. *Birth* **20**: 102–5

Keirse MJNC (1993b) Sexual intercourse for cervical ripening/labour induction. In: Enkin MW, Keirse MJNC, Renfrew MJ, Neilson JP, eds. *Cochrane Database of Systematic Reviews — Pregnancy and Childbirth Module*. Update Software, Oxford: review no 6821

Lucas WE, Anctil AO, Callagan DA (1965) The problem of post-term pregnancy. *Am J Obstet Gynecol* **91**: 241–50

Naeye RL (1978) Causes of perinatal mortality excess in prolonged gestations. *Am J Epidemiol* **108**: 429–33

Neilson JP (1993a) Cardiotocography for antepartum fetal assessment. In: Enkin MW, Keirse MJNC, Renfrew MJ, Neilson JP, eds. *Cochrane Database of Systematic Reviews — Pregnancy and Childbirth Module.* Update Software, Oxford: review no 3881

Neilson JP (1993b) Doppler ultrasound in high risk pregnancies. In: Enkin MW, Keirse MJNC, Renfrew MJ, Neilson JP, eds. *Cochrane Database of Systematic Reviews — Pregancy and Childbirth Module.* Update Software, Oxford: review no 3889

Pearce JM, McParland PJ (1991) A comparison of Doppler flow velocity waveforms, amniotic fluid columns, and the nonstress test as a means of monitoring post-dates pregnancies. *Obstet Gynecol* **77**: 204–8

Royal College of Obstetricians and Gynaecologists Medical Audit Unit (1993) *Effective Procedures in Obstetrics Suitable for Audit.* Royal College of Obstetricians and Gynaecologists, London

Stokes HJ, Newnham JP (1991) Doppler flow velocity waveform analysis in postdate pregnancies. *Aust NZ J Obstet Gynaecol* **31**: 27–30

Walkinshaw S (1993) Biophysical profile scoring: a critical review. In: Neilson J, Chambers S, eds. *Obstetric Ultrasound.* Oxford University Press, Oxford: 151–72

World Health Organisation (1977) *Manual of the International Statistical Classification of Diseases Injuries and Causes of Death.Vol 1.* World Health Organisation, Geneva: 773

8 Management of the first stage of labour

H Gee, K Sharif

The management of delay in labour has been dominated by the use of oxytocin to augment the 'powers' of labour. However, this empirical approach has not been rigorously tested and 'failure to progress' remains a major clinical problem. A return to an analysis of the underlying pathophysiology is advocated.

The 1960s and 1970s saw great interest and optimism in the management of labour. Electronic monitoring technology became cheaper and readily available. The vision of science entering the art of obstetrics was in accord with the times. Now, as stock is taken of the results, there is increasing concern over intervention rates and questions are being asked about the intrusion of technology into what many consider to be a natural process. As a result, there is pressure to move maternity care into the community, including intrapartum care. Controlled trials are not available to directly assess these changes, but indirect evidence has been produced by simulating 'home' conditions within the hospital environment (MacVicar *et al*, 1993). These data show that one-third of low-risk women will require intrapartum transfer to medical care and of these one-third will be for problems associated with progress in labour. Thus, obstetricians have voiced their concerns but the onus is on us to justify our practice. To this end, this paper critically evaluates management policies commonly employed in the first stage of labour.

Two concepts have governed our management of delivery. Firstly, that the duration of labour is proportional to morbidity and mortality. This is undoubtedly true but when progress is delayed is it the duration or the underlying pathology which is causative? Surely it must be the latter. Secondly, that progress is governed primarily by the 'powers' of labour. The other two Ps, the passages and passengers assume secondary importance mainly because the obstetrician has influence over them only via the powers. Obstetricians here fall into the common trap of excluding the possibilities they have not considered.

The corollary of these two concepts is that increasing the powers in prolonged labour will shorten its duration and improve outcome. There may be some evidence for the former but not for the latter.

Active management

Active management offered the prospect of removing poor progress from our delivery suites (Duignan, 1985). However, despite widespread adoption, caesarean section rates have risen in nearly all hospitals and 'failure to progress' has made the largest proportionate contribution (Kiwanuka and Moore, 1987).

Only recently have randomised clinical trials been available. The first study by Lopez-Zeno *et al* (1992) compared aggressive with low-grade oxytocin regimens. A small, statistically non-significant (p= 0.18) reduction in caesarean section rate (10.5% compared to 14.1% was shown by the aggressive regimen which just reached significance after statistical manipulation. Even if this latter figure is accepted, the control should have been a placebo. Interestingly, a bigger reduction in caesarean section rates was seen overall (from 20.9%) presumably from the Hawthorne effect, ie. any intervention will affect outcome. This is why historical controls, which form the basis for most claims to the efficacy of active management should be viewed with scepticism. Two better designed studies by Frigoletto *et al* (1995) and Cammu and Van Eeckhout (1996) show a modest reduction in the duration of labour but no difference in operative delivery rates or neonatal outcome.

So, why should 'failure to progress' continue to plague delivery? There is little or no evidence to suggest the 'passenger' is getting larger and the bony 'passages' are not now subject to pathology arising from nutritional deficiencies which were once commonplace. Where should our attention be focused? How robust are our concepts of normality regarding labour and how reliable are the monitoring techniques on which we base our judgements? Lastly, what are the benefits and side-effects of interventions currently available?

Monitoring

Cervicography

Friedman's meticulous observations on cervical dilatation and descent of the presenting part laid the foundations for current monitoring of labour progress (Friedman, 1967). His division of the first stage of labour into latent and active phases remains standard teaching as does his classification of aberrance into prolonged latent phase, primary dysfunctional labour and secondary arrest. However, the limits of biological variation within any given population have not been established statistically. Thus the cervicogram described by Philpott and Castle (1972) was for use in an African population to determine the appropriate place of delivery. Studd (1973) used this cervicogram on a population in Birmingham UK but had to make pragmatic modifications to prevent inappropriate decision making. No prospective study was performed to verify the assumptions nor to identify the benefits of this monitoring. Beazley and Kurjak (1972) did apply statistical analysis to their population in London, but their action line differentiates 80% and 20% chances of low risk outcome depending on whether progress is above or below the line respectively. It does not differentiate normal from abnormal, nor does it say a particular pattern of progress warrants caesarean section or any other intervention for that matter. The cervicogram is only an aid to the management of labour. It is a sign not a diagnosis. The detection of departure from low risk should raise the awareness of the clinician to the likelihood of pathology in the powers, the response of the passages and the mechanism of transit of the passenger down the birth canal. In other branches of medicine, the treatment of symptoms and signs rather than diagnoses of pathology is scorned, yet it has become the mainstay of delivery suite practise.

Abnormal labour patterns

Prolonged latent phase: The beginning and end of the latent phase are hard to define and different definitions cloud the interpretation of studies. Some would say this phase of labour does not exist. If cervical dilatation is taken as the hallmark of labour then the latent phase would be classified as 'pre-labour'. Nevertheless, particularly in nulliparous women, a time when regular, painful contractions are present and cervical change, albeit subtle, is manifest if looked for carefully, would fulfill the criteria for labour. An incidence 3.5 % in nulliparous labour is to be found. It is less common in multiparous women.

Friedman's original work suggested the latent phase could last up to 20 hours (mean 8.6 hours) in nulliparous women and 14 hours (mean 5.3 hours) in multiparous women. Because the retrospective diagnosis of the onset of labour from the woman's memory may be considered unreliable, others have chosen, purely arbitrarily, the time from admission, resulting in shorter values. The end of the latent phase occurs at the inflexion to more rapid progress which denotes the active phase. This occurs at approximately 3–4 cm.

Retropective identification is easy but not so prospectively.

The definition of the latent phase is not merely academic. True prolongation is associated with increased maternal and neonatal morbidity (Chelmow *et al*, 1993) and the administration of oxytocin to correct poor progress does not yield the desired results. Caesarean section is 10 times more likely and one-third of neonates will have poor Apgar scores (Cardozo *et al*, 1982).

Primary dysfunctional labour: This is defined as an active phase progress rate of less than 1 cm/hr before an active phase slope has been established. Confusion with prolonged latent phase is clearly a danger. This pattern is considered the most common aberrance, affecting 26% of spontaneous nulliparous and 8% multiparous labour. The underlying pathology of this pattern has never been specified. Hypotonic uterine activity must be a major contributor and one which would respond well to oxytocin. Eighty per cent of nulliparous women and 90% of multiparous women will respond. However, other pathologies cannot be excluded. For example, abnormal mechanisms such as persistent occipito-posterior position may affect transmission of forces and the influence of the non-compliant cervix is only now being considered. These pathologies may or may not respond favourably to manipulation of the powers. Non-response carries a 77% chance of caesarean section (Cardozo *et al*, 1982).

Secondary arrest: This occurs when cervical dilatation ceases after a normal portion of active phase dilatation. The pattern is usually associated with cephalopelvic disproportion, either absolute or arising from abnormal mechanism and deflexion of the presenting part. Six per cent of nulliparous women and 2 per cent of multiparous women demonstrate this pattern. Response to oxytocin is variable (Cardozo *et al*, 1982).

A treacherous variant is slow progress over a 7–10 cm.

interval. Oxytocin has little influence but the pattern is associated with instrumental delivery, which is often particularly difficult.

If progress has been normal initially, uterine activity must have been efficient. Further increase in uterine activity in an attempt to improve cervical dilatation must carry the danger of going beyond physiological limits. That is not to say that it will never be of value. If the risks are recognised and the specific aim is to correct an abnormal mechanism or to improve flexion, the intervention may be justified.

Assessment of uterine activity

The technology of the 1970s provided the ability to monitor intrauterine pressure (IUP). This appeared more scientific because it was an objective measurement. However, by the 1980s questions were being raised about its value (Gordon, 1984).

Several units of uterine activity have been devised for clinical practice, namely Montivideo units, Alexandria units, uterine activity integral and mean active pressure. All aim to combine amplitude and repetition frequency, with or without contraction duration and tone, into a single value (Gee and Olah, 1993). The fact that there are so many indicates that none fulfills clinical demands. To some extent this is because IUP is not a simple, independent variable. It is determined not only by myometrial tone but also by the compliance of 'passive' elements within the uterine wall (Coren and Csapo, 1963), the most notable being the cervix (Gee *et al*, 1988). In addition, uterine size will also play a part. For a given wall tension, the smaller uterus will generate more IUP.

Disparities exist between the level of uterine activity found in spontaneous labour and the 'safe' level determined from induced or oxytocin-stimulated labours (Chua *et al*, 1990; Gibb *et al*, 1984). These inconsistencies may relate not so much to the 'power' of uterine activity that a fetus may endure but more to the duration over which it is applied.

Thus high uterine activity in spontaneous labour, when cervical compliance is in keeping with myometrial activity, will result in rapid progress and a short, sustainable period of fetal duress. Conversely, in the face of a non-compliant, non-responding cervix, a fetus subjected to a long period of similar, or even lower uterine activity will succumb to the repeated episodes of reduced placental perfusion which have been demonstrated even during physiological contractions (Janbu and Neshein, 1987).

In clinical practice, IUP monitoring confers no benefit, even in the management of oxytocin stimulated labours, when compared with external guard ring tocodynamometry (Chua *et al*, 1990) which can only truly reflect repetition frequency. This may be so because the predominant effect of oxytocin is reflected in repetition frequency. A contraction rate of three every ten minutes should be adequate, four every ten minutes being the limit.

Interventions

Acceleration/augmentation

These terms have imprecise definitions. 'Acceleration' presumably means returning a slow rate of progress to some notional norm. This is usually achieved by increasing, or 'augmenting', the powers. The terms have almost become synonymous, illustrating the clinicians' compulsive link between the powers and progress.

Oxytocin

This is the most commonly used drug in obstetric practice. It increases the rate of contractions in the quiescent myometrium (Caldeyro-Barcia *et al*, 1957). It slows transmission of electrical activity, thereby improving myometrial coordination. These two properties will improve contractility of a hypotonic myometrium. Delay due to this cause is highly likely to respond favourably because a specific pharmacological remedy is being employed. Whether acceleration in progress leads to better outcome when uterine activity is adequate has yet to be proven.

Escalation of oxytocin when the myometrium is acting optimally produces more rapid contractions, but of lower amplitude, and eventually basal tone rises. Uterine hyper-stimulation is readily apparent in its grossest form (Figure 1) but milder forms can pass unnoticed by clinicians. These effects in combination reduce the recovery time for placental perfusion between contractions, potentially resulting in a cumulative hypoxia and fetal distress.

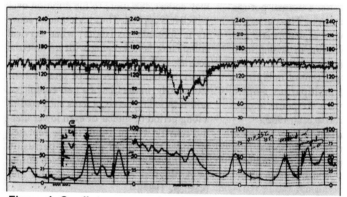

Figure 1. Cardiotocogram showing the effect of oxytocin hyperstimulation. Intrauterine pressure is shown (lower trace). Repetition frequency of the contractions is increased, with a reduction in amplitude above an elevated basal tone. The effect on the fetus is clearly apparent from the fetal heart rate recording (upper trace)

The response of the cervix to oxytocin alters at around 3–4 cms dilatation. Until this time, particularly when effacement has not taken place, contractions rather than dilatation may be observed (Olah *et al*, 1993). They are associated with prolongation of the latent phase and are more common in oxytocin-stimulated labours. Administration of oxytocin in the latent phase is associated, in retrospective studies (Cardozo *et al, 1982;* Chelmow *et al*, 1993), with poor response and increased morbidity. The diagnosis of the transition from latent to active phase is crucial.

Amniotomy

Much debate has taken place over the benefits of this practice. In terms of releasing prostaglandins for their effect on the myometrium and cervix, there are potential advantages. Clinical trials suggest that its effects are marginal. There does appear to be a shortening of the duration of labour but no improvement in outcome (UK Amniotomy Group, 1994).

Amniotomy to examine the liquor for meconium is of dubious clinical value. Few would advocate intervention for meconium alone if the cardiotocogram (CTG) was normal. Amnio-infusion, whereby saline is infused into the amniotic cavity to correct oligohydramnios, has shown benefits by reducing the incidence of heart rate irregularities, operative intervention and meconium aspiration. These data suggest that releasing the liquor can be deleterious. Amniotomy may be necessary to gain access to the fetus for internal CTG monitoring, fetal electocardiogram analysis, oximetry or pH measurement. These are valid reasons but would only be indicated in high-risk cases.

Posture

This has been considered to alter progress in labour. During the first stage of labour the uterus acts as an isometric system, particularly when the membranes are intact. Theoretically, maternal position should have little effect on such a system. In practice, however, ambulation during the first stage has been associated with shorter labour, use of fewer narcotic analgesics and less need for oxytocin augmentation when compared with the supine position. Moreover, vena caval compression in the supine position is well recognised and should be avoided. Epidural analgesia is now a standard practice in most units with a 25–30% uptake. Labouring women should not be denied access to this form of analgesia which by any standards is remarkably effective. However, its limitation of maternal mobility during labour and long-term after-effects (MacArthur *et al*, 1991), such as backache, must be acknowledged.

Complex labour

As caesarean section becomes more common, the clinician is more likely to be faced with the management of labour in a woman with a scarred uterus. The dictum 'once a section, always a section' has been abandoned even in the USA. The incidence of uterine rupture in lower uterine segment incisions is low (0.3–0.7%). Vaginal delivery can be expected in two-thirds of cases.

IUP monitoring has been advocated as a means of reducing the likelihood of over-tensioning the scar. However, theoretical considerations and clinical observations (Beckley *et al*, 1991) indicate that there are no such safeguards and the association of poor progress and apparently poor uterine activity using IUP measurement due to the effect of the deficient scar can lead to the inappropriate use of oxytocin. Selection of cases and the exclusion of true cephalopelvic disproportion are crucial. Poor progress should always be viewed with caution. Other warning signs such as fetal heart rate abnormalities and antepartum haemorrhage, must be sought. Only when hypotonic uterine activity is held to be the only pathology may oxytocin be administered with caution. Contraction repetition frequency, which may be determined merely by palpation, should be the yardstick.

by H Gee, K Sharif

Paradoxes of labour

So far the assumption has been accepted that progress is related to the powers. However, there are paradoxes to be observed in everyday practice (Gee and Olah, 1993). Multiparous women progress more rapidly than nulliparous women, but do so with lower rates of uterine activity. Conversely, high uterine activity may be associated with poor progress, conditionsthat are often associated with fetal distress. Precipitate labour demonstrates low/normal uterine activity. In preterm labour contractions may be present without progress and delivery, while at the other end of the spectrum delivery can occur with the mother appreciating little uterine activity. These observations suggest that in both physiological and pathological states progress is not only the product of the powers.

Influence of the cervix

The cervix forms part of the uterine wall. Wall tension will be the resultant of myometrial tension and cervical compliance. Thus cervical compliance will determine both the resistance to delivery and uterine activity. As compliance rises, dilatation increases while wall tension and uterine activity fall, in keeping with the paradoxes given above.

The connective tissue structure of the cervix is un-questionable, but that it is a passive structure, dilating in direct response to an active myometrium, is far from the truth. Marked biochemical changes take place over relatively short timescales prior to and during labour. Structural glyco-proteins such as dermatan sulphate, which glue together the collagen fibres, are removed and heparan sulphate, which has low affinity for collagen increases, acting as a 'filler' and allowing dispersion of the collagen. There is a marked peak in hyaluronic acid, which carries with it water, during the latent phase when effacement is taking place (Osmers *et al*, 1993). These changes, even without collagen degradation

99

which is still a controversial issue, alter the character or 'ripeness' of the cervix which becomes more deformable and compliant. Abnormal glycoprotein composition of the cervix has been associated with aberrent progress in labour (Granström *et al*, 1991).

Recording of cervical response to myometrial activity on a contraction cycle-by-cycle basis has demonstrated that dilatation is not directly proportional to the myometrial activity. Measurement of head: cervix pressures and forces has also shown that cervical dilatation is not merely a simple stretching (Gee, 1982; Gough *et al*, 1990). Exactly how efface-ment, dilatation and redistribution of the tissue in the 'taking up' of the cervix are achieved remains enigmatic.

The phenomenon of cervical contractions has already been alluded to. The smooth muscle content of the cervix is small and hitherto has been considered insignificant in functional terms. Recordings of electrical activity (Pajntar *et al*, 1987) from the cervix indicate that these are true contractions. Whether these are a pregnancy function, counterbalancing myometrial activity, carried over into labour or whether they are instrumental in effecting cervical change is unclear.

When induction of labour is to be undertaken, cervical state is taken into consideration. Nothing clearly demarcates the pregnancy uterus from the pre-labour and intrapartum uterus yet our thinking is compartmentalised. A better understanding of the mechanisms which control cervical state could provide pharmacological means to complement control over the powers to determine progress, but with the added attraction that forces on the fetus could be reduced. Prostaglandins are obvious candidates but agents which have little or no utero-tonic effect would be even more attractive. Relaxin, oestrogens and cytokines have potential.

Conclusion

Current labour management does not solve all clinical problems. When policy fails, clinicians often ask whether it has been implemented correctly rather than questioning the policy itself. Unfortunately, many of our labour ward policies are based on convention rather than objective scientific testing. Having said this, policies may have to be adhered to until better alternatives are demonstrated. The deficiencies of current policies, while frustrating to those who implement them, should be the stimulus to further research. Identifying the problem is the first step to finding a solution.

Key points

- The benefits of 'active management' have not been established by controlled clinical trials.
- Control of the 'powers' of labour has not solved the problem of failure to progress in labour.
- The 'resistant' forces to delivery should be given more consideration.
- The importance of cervical state is recognised at induction of labour but not during labour.

References

Beazley JM, Kurjak A (1972) Influence of a partogram on the active management of labour. *Lancet* **2**: 348–51

Beckley S, Gee H, Newton JR (1991) The place of intra-uterine pressure monitoring in the management of scar rupture in labour. *Br J Obstet Gynaecol* **98**: 265–9

Caldeyro-Barcia R, Sica-Blanco Y, Poseiro JJ, Gonzalez-Panizza U, Mendez Bauer C, Alvarez H, Pose SV, Hendricks CH (1957) A quantitative study of the action of synthetic oxytocin on the pregnant human uterus. *J Pharm Exp Ther* **121**: 18–31

Cammu H, Van-Eeckhout E (1996) A randomised controlled trial of early versus delayed use of amniotomy and oxytocin infusion in nulliparous labour. *Br J Obstet Gynaecol* **103**(4): 313–318

Cardozo L, Gibb DMF, Studd JWW, Vasant RV, Cooper DJ (1982) Predictive value of cervimetric patterns in primigravidae. *Br J Obstet Gynaecol* **89**: 33–8

Cardozo L, Pearce JM (1991) Oxytocin in active-phase abnormalities of labour: a randomised study. *Obstet Gynecol* **75**: 152–157

Chelmow D, Kilpatrick SJ, Laros RK (1993) Maternal and neonatal outcomes after prolonged latent phase. *Obstet Gynecol* **81**: 486–91

Chua S, Kurup A, Arulkumaran S, Ratman SS (1990) Augmentation of labor: does internal tocography result in better obstetric outcome than external tocography? *Obstet Gynecol* **76**: 164–7

Coren, RL, Csapo, AI (1963) The intra-amniotic pressure. *Am J Obstet Gynecol* **85**: 470–83

Duignan, N (1985). Active management of labour. In: Studd J ed. *The Management of Labour*. Blackwell Scientific Publications, Oxford: 99

Friedman EA (1967) *Labor: Clinical Evaluation and Management*. Meredith, New York

Frigoletto FD, Lieberman E, Lang JM et al (1995) A clinical trial of active management of labour. *N Engl J Med*, **133** (12): 745–750

Gee H (1982) Uterine activity and cervical resistance determining cervical change in labour. MD Thesis, University of Liverpool, UK

Gee H, Olah KS (1993) Failure to progress in labour. In: Studd J, ed. *Progress in Obstetrics and Gynaecology, Vol 10*. Churchill Livingstone, London: 159–81

Gee H, Taylor EW, Hancox R (1988) A model for the generation of intra-uterine pressure in the human parturient uterus which demonstrates the critical role of the cervix. *J Theor Biol* **133**: 281–91

Gibb DMF, Arulkumaran S, Lun KC, Ratman SS (1984) Characteristics of uterine activity in nulliparous labour. *Br J Obstet Gynaecol* **89**: 220–7

Gordon AJ (1984) Measurement of uterine activity — a useful tool? *Br J Obstet Gynaecol* **91**: 209–10

Gough GW, Randall NJ, Dut G, Sutherland IA, Steer PJ (1990) Head to cervix forces and their relationship to the outcome of labor. *Obstet Gynecol* **75**: 613–8

Granström L, Ekman G, Malmström A (1991) Insufficient remodelling of the uterine connective tissue in women with protracted labour. *Br J Obstet Gynaecol* **98**: 1212– 16

Janbu T, Neshein B (1987) Uterine artery blood velocities during contractions in pregnancy and labour related to intra-uterine pressure. *Br J Obstet Gynaecol* **94**: 1150–5

Kiwanuka AI, Moore WMO (1987) The changing incidence of caesarean section in the health district of central Manchester. *Br J Obstet Gynaecol* **94**: 440–4

Lopez-Zeno JA, Peaceman AM, Adashek JA, Socol ML (1992) A controlled trial of a program for the active management of labor. *N Engl J Med* **326**: 450–4

MacArthur C, Lewis M, Knox EG (1991) *Health after Childbirth*. HMSO, London

MacVicar J, Dobbie G, Owen-Johnstone L, Jagger C, Hopkins M, Kennedy J (1993) Simulated home delivery in hospital: a randomised controlled trial. *Br J Obstet Gynaecol* **100**: 316–23

Olah KS, Gee H, Brown JS (1993) Cervical contractions: the response of the cervix to oxytocic stimulation in the latent phase of labour. *Br J Obstet Gynaecol* **100**: 635–40

Osmers R, Rath W, Pflanz MA, Kuhn W, Stuhlsatz H, Szeverenyi M (1993) Glycosaminoglycans in cervical connective tissue during pregnancy and parturition. *Obstet Gynecol* **81**: 88–92

Pajntar M, Roskar E, Rudel D (1987) Electromyographic observations on the human cervix during delivery. *Am J Obstet Gynecol* **156**: 691–7

Philpott RH, Castle WM (1972) Cervicographs in the management of labour in primigravidae: I. The alert line for detecting abnormal labour. *J Obstet Gynaecol Br Emp* **79**: 592–98

UK Amniotomy Group (1994) A multicentre randomised trial of amniotomy in spontaneous first labour at term. *Br J Obstet Gynaecol* **101**: 307–9

9 Assisted reproduction techniques

SV Jones

Many couples with infertility will require a form of assisted reproduction to achieve a pregnancy. Assisted reproduction techniques, including intrauterine insemination, gamete intrafallopian transfer and in-vitro fertilisation, are considered in this review.

Increasingly large numbers of couples are seeking help in achieving a pregnancy, although there is no evidence that the prevalence of infertility has changed over the last 10 years (Templeton *et al*, 1991). It is estimated that 14% of married couples suffer from involuntary infertility, and this figure increases to 25% in the 35–39-year-old group (Soules, 1988). This has obvious implications at a time when many couples are postponing starting a family until their 30s. It is estimated that about 25% of these couples will require assisted reproduction techniques (ARTs).

For ARTs to be effective, accurate diagnosis and appropriate therapy is required. Detailed history taking and examination coupled with appropriate investigation is therefore mandatory for success. In-vitro fertilisation (IVF) was initially developed to bypass damaged or occluded fallopian tubes, but has developed to become the treatment of choice for other causes of infertility. The two other main ARTs are gamete intrafallopian transfer (GIFT) and intrauterine insemination (IUI) with super-ovulation. The indications for each of these methods are considered below. A number of modifications of these basic techniques are performed.

Drugs used in treatment

A variety of drug treatments are commonly used in ARTs.

Antioestrogens

The most commonly used antioestrogen is clomiphene citrate, but tamoxifen and cyclofenil (now discontinued) have a similar mode of action and are sometimes used.

Clomiphene citrate was first used as an ovulatory stimulant in 1961 and is still the first line of drug treatment for anovulation. It acts on both the hypothalamus and pituitary, increasing the frequency of luteinising hormone releasing hormone (LHRH) pulses released from the hypothalamus, while also increasing the receptivity of the pituitary cells to the LHRH pulses. The combined effect of these actions is an increased release of follicle-stimulating hormone (FSH) and luteinising hormone (LH) from the pituitary, which stimulate ovarian follicular development. There may also be a minor direct effect on the ovary, making it more sensitive to FSH stimulation.

The lowest effective dose of clomiphene should be used, because of its side-effects. This dose is normally 50 mg daily for days 2–6 of the cycle, increasing to 100 mg daily after 1 month if the patient remains anovulatory. If ovulation still fails to occur there is no further benefit in increasing the dose, but 100 mg should be continued for two or three more cycles as some patients do not ovulate on the initial dose but do so subsequently. Side-effects include thickening of cervical mucus (making sperm penetration more difficult), vaginal dryness, hot flushes, ovarian cyst formation, bloating, breast discomfort, nausea and skin rash. Very rarely blurred vision occurs, in which case treatment should be stopped. Twin pregnancies occur in about 5% of cases (about four times higher than in natural conception), but clomiphene is rarely associated with triplet or higher order pregnancies. Miscarriage is more common with clomiphene-induced pregnancies, presumably as a result of increased LH secretion (especially in polycystic ovary patients), but there is no evidence of an increased risk of fetal abnormality.

Human menopausal gonadotrophin (hMG)

hMG is prepared by extracting FSH and LH from the urine of postmenopausal women, and has been in use since the 1960s. It is currently available in several preparations, the most widely used of which contain FSH 75 iu and LH 75 iu.

hMG is administered by intramuscular injection and has a direct stimulatory effect on the ovary to induce follicular development. The patient response to hMG needs to be monitored carefully as the dividing line between inadequate and excessive stimulation can be narrow. hMG can be used to promote single follicular development in anovulatory women (with clomiphene-resistant ovaries) and patients undergoing IUI, but is most often employed to promote multiple follicular development in IVF and GIFT programmes.

Another hMG preparation attempts to mimic the body's natural ratio of gonadotrophins and is presented as ampoules containing FSH 75 iu and LH 25 iu. Preparations containing FSH alone are also available and may be of use in patients with elevated LH levels. The original FSH-only preparation has now been superseded by a highly purified version which can be administered subcutaneously. Synthetic FSH and LH preparations will soon be available as a result of recombinant DNA technology.

hMG may be associated with local inflammatory reactions at the site of injection, and systemic arthralgia and fever have been reported. However, the serious side-effects of hMG treatment are multiple pregnancy and ovarian hyperstimulation syndrome (OHSS).

Gonadotrophin releasing hormone (GnRH) analogues

Most units employ pituitary down-regulation as part of the superovulation programme. Spontaneous LH release from the pituitary can interfere with oocyte development and can induce ovulation before oocyte collection. These problems can be overcome by pituitary desensitisation, which also allows scheduling of oocyte collection to avoid unsocial hours.

Long protocol regimens are most commonly used. A GnRH analogue is commenced either on day 2 of the menstrual cycle or in the mid-luteal phase, and hMG is commenced 2–3 weeks later after down-regulation has been confirmed. In the short protocol regimens, a GnRH analogue and hMG are started in the early follicular phase. It may be possible to reduce the initial dose of hMG in the short regimen as there is an initial agonistic 'flare' effect after commencing treatment with a GnRH analogue (Fleming and Coutts, 1990).

Many GNRH analogues are now available and are administered nasally or as a subcutaneous injection. Compounds in most common use are buserelin, nafarelin, goserelin and leuprorelin. The most common side-effects arise from the pseudo-menopausal state induced by the treatment, ie. hot flushes, sweats and mood swings. Headaches are also common, as is sneezing following nasal administration. Rarely, hypersensitive skin rashes occur and treatment should be withdrawn in these cases.

Human chorionic gonadotrophin (hCG)

hCG is obtained from the urine of pregnant women and has a similar action to pituitary LH. It is used in various ways in ARTs. During IUI it is given in ovulatory doses (usually 10 000 iu) when a dominant follicle is ripe (see below) followed by insemination 34–39 hours later; it is also given in subovulatory doses (usually 5000iu) to promote oocyte maturation in IVF and GIFT programmes before egg collection. hCG can also be used to provide luteal support following embryo transfer in IVF programmes where pituitary down-regulation has been employed, but may be associated with an increased incidence of OHSS. Many units now use only progesterone for luteal support.

Techniques

IUI

IUI differs from artificial insemination (by husband or donor) in that prepared sperm is used in a stimulated cycle and this sperm is deposited into the uterine cavity and not the vagina and/or cervix.

Monitoring of the stimulated cycle allows insemination to be timed to coincide with ovulation, as hCG can be given when a follicle reaches 18–19 mm and the insemination performed 34–39 hours later. The sperm is prepared in two ways before insemination. It is first washed (to reduce the risk of infection as the cervical mucus barrier is bypassed) and then subjected to a 'swim up' technique which enables only those sperm most likely to be capable of fertilisation to be used for the insemination.

The indications for IUI (Table 1) include cervical mucus defects/dysfunction, unexplained infertility and borderline male infertility. In cases of severe male factor problems, IUI with donor sperm is very successful, but in borderline cases using partners' sperm, the results are less encouraging, especially if the 'swim up' sample contains less than one million sperm (Horvath *et al*, 1989).

The major complication of stimulated cycle IUI is overstimulation, ie. the production of several follicles which may result in a high order pregnancy if treatment is continued, or the development of OHSS. Thus ultrasound monitoring of ovarian response is crucial, and treatment should be abandoned (and the patient advised to contracept) or converted to another ART (IVF, IVC or GIFT) if more than three or four large follicles are present.

Table 1. Indications for choice of treatment	
Intrauterine insemination	Unexplained infertility
	Cervical mucus dysfunction/hostility
	? Borderline male infertility
Gamete intrafallopian transfer	Unexplained infertility
	Cervical mucus dysfunction/hostility
	Endometriosis with patent tubes
In-vitro fertilisation	Tubal damage
	Unexplained infertility when other treatments have failed
	Endometriosis
	Male factor (+/- micromanipulation techniques)
	Multifactorial
	Ovarian failure using donated oocytes

GIFT

GIFT can be very successful in well-chosen patients. Suitable patients should have patent tubes and a diagnosis of unexplained infertility, cervical mucus defects or dysfunction, mild or moderate degrees of endometriosis, or borderline male factor problems.

Table 2. Assisted reproduction techniques: advantages and disadvantages		
	Advantages	**Disadvantages**
Intrauterine insemination	Minimally invasive	Fertilisation not confirmed
	Less emotional commitment	Tubes must be patent
	Less expensive	Lower success rates
	Less time-consuming	Risk of high multiple pregnancy
Gamete intrafallopian transfer	Natural environment for fertilisation	Fertilisation not confirmed
	Less technically demanding embryologically	Tubes must be patent
		GA and laparoscopy required
		Expensive
In-vitro fertilisation	Fertilisation confirmed	Emotionally demanding
	Best success rates	Technically demanding
	Can be used for most categories of infertility	Expensive
GA = general anaesthetic		

The technique involves pituitary desensitisation and ovarian stimulation as for IVF (see below), but eggs are recovered by laparoscopy and the oocytes are identified and graded by the embryologist. Prepared sperm is then drawn into a fine catheter together with three of the best oocytes obtained and the catheter is passed into the fallopian tube. The sperm–egg mixture is then deposited within the tube, usually two eggs on one side and one on the other.

If facilities are available, excess oocytes are also mixed with sperm, both as a diagnostic aid to confirm fertilisation and also as a therapeutic aid, as the resulting embryos can be frozen for subsequent treatment.

Complications associated with GIFT are essentially those associated with IVF (see below), although there are the additional complications of laparoscopy (Table 2).

IVF

The first birth after IVF treatment was in 1978 (Steptoe and Edwards, 1978) following laparoscopic oocyte retrieval of a single egg during a natural cycle (ie. with no ovarian stimulation). This was the culmination of many years research and IVF has now become a simpler and more successful treatment as a result of three major advances, namely superovulation, transvaginal ultrasound-guided oocyte retrieval and pituitary down-regulation. IVF has an advantage over other ARTs in that diagnostic information about the fertilisation potential of the sperm is obtained, and the treatment is effective. Success rates are shown in Figure 1.

Treatment cycle

There are six major steps in an IVF treatment cycle:

Pituitary down-regulation: Most units now employ down-regulation as part of IVF treatment. This is achieved by the use of a GnRH analogue (see above). Down-regulation allows precise control of the treatment cycle and also prevents ovulation occurring before oocyte retrieval by suppressing the endogenous LH surge.

Ovarian stimulation: Multiple follicular growth is encouraged in most IVF treatments as transfer of more than one embryo (together with embryo freezing and subsequent

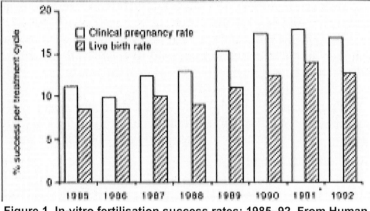

Figure 1. In-vitro fertilisation success rates: 1985–92. From Human Fertilisation and Embryology Authority (1994). *Figures for August–December

thaw-replacement cycles) improves success rates, although some natural cycle IVF is still performed.

Stimulation is achieved by the use of the gonadotrophins discussed above. Ovarian response can be monitored ultrasonographically (Figure 2) and by oestradiol measurements (serum or urine), and needs to be tailored to the individual to ensure an adequate response while avoiding OHSS (see below).

Figure 2. Vaginal ultrasound scan of a human menopausal gonadotrophin stimulated ovary

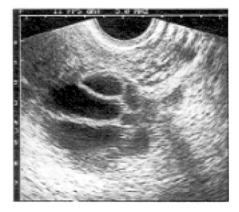

Response is considered adequate when the largest follicle is 16–20 mm average diameter with several other follicles greater than 14 mm. hCG is then administered to promote final oocyte maturation before egg recovery 34–36 hours later.

Oocyte retrieval: Vaginal ultrasound scanning has enabled oocyte retrieval to be performed on an outpatient basis, and can be performed without general anaesthesia. A needle guide is attached to the scan probe, allowing direct puncture of the follicles with a fine gauge needle passed through the vaginal fornix (Figure 3). The follicular fluid is then aspirated into test tubes and handed to the embryologist for oocyte identification and grading.

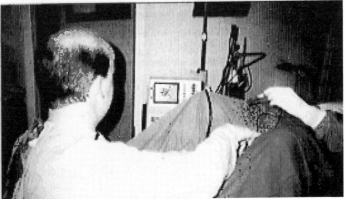

Figure 3. Transvaginal ultrasound-guided oocyte recovery

Transvaginal oocyte retrieval has largely superseded the laparoscopic method because it is simple and highly effective, which patients prefer. Complications are rare, but include perforation of abdominal viscera (especially blood vessels) and infection.

IVF: Following oocyte recovery the eggs are transferred to a nutrient culture medium. The partner's sperm is prepared in a similar way to that in IUI, and the eggs are inseminated 40 hours after the time of the hCG administration. About 100,000 motile sperm are added to each egg and fertilisation awaited. If fertilisation is successful, two pronuclei are seen after 12–18 hours and subsequently cleavage and cell division occurs.

Recent developments in micromanipulation techniques have enabled the fertilisation of eggs by single sperms, thus allowing treatment in cases of severe male factor infertility. Intracytoplasmic sperm injection involves fixing an oocyte by suction to a holding pipette and picking up a single sperm in a sharpened micropipette, which is then injected directly into the oocyte under microscope control. Excellent fertilisation rates can be obtained by experienced operators.

Embryo transfer: A maximum of three embryos (Figure 4) are replaced about 48 hours after egg collection, when they are usually at the 2- to 8-cell stage. Embryo transfer is a straightforward proce-dure involving the passage of a fine catheter containing the embryos transcervically and deposition of the embryos into the uterine cavity.

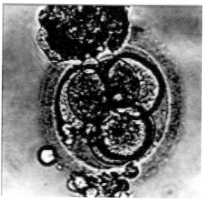

Luteal support: As a consequence of pituitary down-regulation there is little or no endogenous hormonal support for the luteal phase. This support

Figure 4. Embryos in vitro

can be provided by the administration of exogenous hCG or progesterone.

Pregnancy testing is performed 2 weeks after embryo trans-fer and ultrasound scanning is then performed on days 35 and 50.

The major complications of IVF are multiple pregnancy and OHSS. With a limit of three embryos being transferred, high-order multiple pregnancies are extremely rare, but even triplet pregnancies are associated with a very significant increase in perinatal morbidity and mortality, as well as socioeconomic difficulties for parents, and should be avoided.

OHSS is a potentially fatal side-effect of any ovulatory stimulant and is a complex syndrome associated with ovarian enlargement, ascites and hypovolaemia in its most severe form (Table 3). There are less severe degrees of OHSS: in its mildest form it can be treated conservatively on an outpatient basis by encouraging rest, oral fluids and analgesia. However, anything other than the mildest form needs admission to a unit with intensive care facilities and with staff experienced in its management on hand.

Gamete donation

The role of donated sperm is well established, and excellent results can be achieved in cases of severe male factor infertility using donor sperm either as a straightforward insemination, or with mild super-ovulation and IUI as well as GIFT and IVF.

Oocyte donation is obviously more difficult than sperm donation, but a number of centres are now offering this service. It is indicated for women with ovulatory failure, either primary (eg. Turner's syndrome) or secondary (premature ovarian failure), for women who have had their ovaries surgically removed, for women unresponsive to gonadotrophins, and for women with genetic disorders to prevent transmission to the offspring. Oocytes are obtainedfrom donors, many of whom donate for altruistic reasons, but donors are also recruited from other sources, eg. women undergoing sterilisation or 'free' IVF where a proportion ofthe eggs are donated and a portion are kept for their own treatment.

Table 3. Ovarian hyperstimulation syndrome (OHSS)	
Risk factors for OHSS	Polycystic ovarian syndrome
	Young
	Thin
	High oestradiol
	Pregnancy
	Use of exogenous human chorionic gonadotrophin
	Use of gonadotrophin releasing hormone analogues
OHSS is associated with	Increased ovarian size
	Ascites
	Hypovolaemia
	Haemoconcentration
	Hypotension
	Renal failure
	Thromboembolic phenomena
	Adult respiratory distress syndrome
Therapy is supportive and based on monitoring	Fluid and electrolyte balance
	Liver function and clotting parameters
	Ultrasound: ovaries and ascites
	Plasma and urine osmolarity
There is no specific treatment, although intravenous albumin given prophylactically may help prevent the development of OHSS.	

Key points

- Assisted conception offers the most effective treatment in about 25% of cases of infertility.
- Assisted reproduction techniques include intrauterine insemination, gamete intrafallopian transfer and in-vitro fertilisation (IVF).
- IVF has an advantage over other techniques as fertilisation is confirmed.
- Efficient investigation and accurate diagnosis are vital to ensure correct therapy and obtain good success rates.
- Patient counselling and support are prerequisites to successful therapy.

References

Fleming R, Coutts JRT (1990) Induction of multiple follicular development for IVF. *Br Med Bull* **46**: 596–615

Horvath PM, Bohrer M, Shelden RM, Kemmann E (1989) The relationship of sperm parameters to cycle fecundity in superovulated women undergoing IUI. *Fertil Steril* **52**: 288–94

Human Fertilisation and Embryology Authority (1994) HFEA 3rd Annual Report. HFEA, London

Soules MR (1988) Prevention of infertility. *Fertil Steril* **49**: 582–4

Steptoe PC, Edwards RG (1978) Birth after the reimplantation of a human embryo. *Lancet* **ii**: 366

Templeton A, Fraser C, Thompson B (1991) Infertility — epidemiology and referrral practice. *Hum Reprod* **6**: 1391–4

10 Endometrial resection

RJ Armatage, RG Farquharson

Transcervical resection of the endometrium (TCRE) is a technique that has gained popularity in gynaecological practice as an alternative to hysterectomy for patients presenting with menstrual disturbances. The advantages of such a technique over traditional hysterectomy include shorter hospital stay, more rapid recovery allowing return to normal daily activity and reduced perioperative morbidity, with associated health and economic benefits.

Menorrhagia is a common and debilitating condition and patients with this disorder frequently present to GPs and gynaecologists. The annual frequency of GP consultation for this condition is 31 per 1000 women (*Morbidity Statistics from General Practice 1981–1982,* 1986). Drug therapy may provide temporary relief of symptoms, but these usually return when medication is stopped. Compliance is often poor due to side effects of the drugs used, and some therapies can only be recommended in the short term. Failure of medical treatment invariably leads to surgical management.

Until recently, hysterectomy has been the only surgical option and remains the mainstay of management. In 1985, a total of 18600 hysterectomies were performed in England to alleviate menstrual disorders. This represented over 650 hospital beds occupied every day (*Hospital Inpatient Enquiry,* 1985).

Several minimally invasive surgical techniques, including transcervical resection of the endometrium (TCRE), endometrial ablation by neodymium-yttrium aluminium garnet (Nd-YAG) laser and radiofrequency-induced thermal ablation, have been developed as alternatives to hysterectomy for the operative treatment of menorrhagia. This article concentrates on endometrial resection which, in comparison with ablation of the endometrium, has the additional advantage of providing tissue for histological examination.

Brief history of hysteroscopy

The first use of the 'hysteroscope' was described by Pantaleoni in 1869, who used it to identify and cauterise an endometrial polyp. With the aid of improved light sources and optical systems, diagnostic hysteroscopy became an accepted, although not widely practised, technique by the 1970s. Realisation of the potential for the therapeutic use of the hysteroscope grew after Neuwirth and Amin's (1976) description of the hysteroscopic electro-surgical excision and removal of pedunculated submucous fibroids. However, it was not until 1983 that DeCherney and Polan first used a urological resectoscope for the emergency treatment of intractable uterine bleeding in a series of 11 patients who were deemed unfit for hysterectomy. The technique was further developed in France by Hamou and later refined by Magos *et al* in England who coined the term TCRE (Magos *et al*, 1989).

Patient selection for TCRE

The treatment criteria for TCRE are listed in Table 1. Successful outcomes are more likely to be achieved if these criteria are strictly applied in every case. Thorough counselling with regard to the risks of the procedure, the expected reduction in menstrual flow (which may not become apparent for 3–4 months) and the risk of pregnancy is essential before TCRE.

The long-term effects of this relatively new procedure are presently unknown. There is a theoretical risk of endometrial carcinoma occurring in residual islands of endometrium, even in those patients who become amenorrhoeic as a result of surgery. For this reason, combined hormone replacement therapy should be prescribed for those who subsequently desire oestrogen supplementation.

Table 1. Treatment criteria for transcervical resection of the endometrium
Menstrual distrubances warranting hysterectomy
Benign endometrial pathology
Failure of medical treatment
Uterine size smaller than the equivalent of a 12-week pregnancy
Submucous fibroids <10 cm diameter
Completed family
Absence of other gynaecological conditions (eg. ovarian cyst, endometriosis, pelvic inflammatory disease)

Preparation of the endometrium before TCRE

The aim of TCRE is to resect the endometrium to just beyond the basal epithelium to prevent endometrial regeneration. Since the endometrial thickness varies throughout the menstrual cycle, one would expect to achieve better results if TCRE were performed early in the follicular phase of the menstrual cycle or after thinning of the endometrium with drugs such as progestogens, danazol or gonadotrophin-releasing hormone (GnRH) analogues (eg. Zoladex).

A study comparing the efficacy of danazol and Zoladex in producing endometrial atrophy before TCRE did not show any significant difference between the drugs, although the GnRH analogue was better tolerated (Ewen *et al*, 1994). A randomised trial assessing the influence of Zoladex *vs* no endometrial preparation on the outcome of TCRE showed no significant difference in the rates of amenorrhoea in the long term (MacDonald *et al*, 1994). Our results in patients who did not receive endometrial thinning agents support this view and are comparable with those of other centres (see below).

Operative technique

Day case treatment is almost universally practised, with the advantage of early resumption to normal activity.

Intrauterine endoscopic surgery requires a 26 FG continuous flow resectoscope with a 4 mm forward-oblique telescope and a 24 FG cutting loop connected to a power unit that is capable of blending both cutting and coagulating currents. Distention of the uterine cavity is essential for providing a panoramic view of the uterine cavity, including the fundus and tubal ostia. The operator must orientate him/herself before resecting any tissue in order to minimise the risk of perforation of the uterus and concomitant damage to structures outside the uterus. Glycine 1.5%, a non-essential amino acid solution, is a poor conductor of electricity and therefore a suitable distention medium. If the reservoir is placed between 80 and 100 cm above the level of the uterus, sufficient pressure is created to adequately distend the uterine cavity. Problems relating to glycine delivery include too low a pressure, where an inadequate view is obtained, and too high a pressure, where the distention medium is forced into the circulation via veins in the myometrium, thus causing fluid overload.

Tubing is connected to the exhaust port of the resectoscope to allow continuous drainage of glycine by gravity into a calibrated receptacle. By maintaining a continuous flow of glycine through the cavity, a clear view is obtained at all times. Mechanical irrigation pumps specifically designed for this purpose are available, but only add to the cost rather than the safety of the operation.

Resectoscopes may be fitted with either active or passive handle mechanisms. We prefer the active mechanism where the cutting loop is exposed at rest. When introducing the resectoscope into the uterine cavity, the loop needs to be withdrawn into the outer sheath of the resectoscope to avoid damage to the loop. Once inside the cavity with the glycine flowing, the operator needs to orientate him/herself with respect to the tubal ostia, the fundus and the length/size of the cavity. At this point, the cutting loop can be released to approximately 1.5–2cm in front of the end of the resectoscope.

Starting on the posterior wall at the fundus of the cavity, strips of endometrium are cut, creating furrows along the entire length of the cavity by slowly withdrawing the resectoscope while keeping the end of the cutting loop in sight at all times (Figure 1a). On reaching the level of the internal cervical os, identified by the appearance of a paler epithelium, the loop may be withdrawn into the outer sheath, thus trapping the length of resected endometrium which may then be removed immediately so as not to obstruct the view of future cuts. This process is then repeated systematically around the entire cavity until all of the endometrium has been removed.

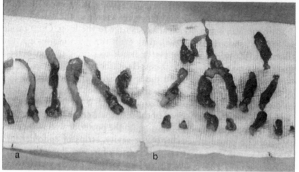

Figure 1. 'Strips' (a) and 'chips' (b) of resected endometrium available for histological assessment

An alternative technique of resecting small 'chips' of endometrium has been described, with the chips being removed at the end of the procedure by suction or curettage

(Figure 1b). Special care is required when resecting tissue at the uterine fundus and around the tubal ostia, where the myometrium is thinnest, and this is often best achieved using a forward-angled loop. All resected tissue should be sent for histological examination.

Having completed the resection phase of the procedure, the cutting loop is replaced by a rollerball coagulator. The cavity should be inspected and any residual islands of endometrium diathermised. By reducing the flow rate of glycine, any bleeding vessels can be identified and coagulated to secure haemostasis.

Complications of TCRE

These are summarised in Table 2.

Uterine perforation

Uterine perforation is an infrequent complication with an incidence of between 0.46% and 4%, depending on the experience of the operator (Magos *et al*, 1991; Pyper and Haeri, 1991; Rankin and Steinberg, 1992; Dwyer *et al*, 1993). Characteristically, this is recognised by a sudden loss of view as the cavity walls collapse and the distention media is rapidly lost into the abdominal cavity. This may be treated conservatively where perforation is known to have been caused by the resectoscope alone, but laparoscopy and/or laparotomy should be performed in all cases where perforation occurred during the use of electrosurgery.

Fluid overload

This much publicised and potentially fatal complication of TCRE may result when more than 1300 ml of glycine is absorbed into the circulation (van Herendael, 1993). Glycine in iso-osmotic concentration can cause haemodilution, extra-cellular volume expansion and hyponatraemia.

Hyperammonaemia may also occur as a result of the rapid metabolism of glycine. High ammonia concentrations in the central nervous system alter neural amino acid metabolism, resulting in the production of false neurotransmitters, causing encephalopathy.

Frequent fluid balance measurements during and at the end of surgery are therefore imperative. Surgery should be abandoned in cases where there is a negative balance of more than 1000 ml.

Table 2. Potential complications following transcervical endometrial resection		
Intraoperative		Uterine perforation
		Fluid overload
		Primary haemorrhage
		Technical failure — eg. cervical stenosis
Postoperative	Short term	Infection
		Secondary haemorrhage
		Haematometra
		Adenomyosis
		Treatment failure
	Long term	Recurrence of symptoms
		Pregnancy
		Uterine malignancy

Primary haemorrhage

This complication rarely occurs where the depth of resection is limited to the superficial myometrium. Troublesome bleeding may be encountered in the isthmic portion of the uterus which contains a rich plexus of veins. Where coagulation with the rollerball is not sufficient to secure haemostasis, tamponade obtained by inserting a 30 ml Foley catheter balloon into the uterine cavity for 4 hours is usually effective.

Haematometra and adenomyosis

The exact incidence of haematometra after TCRE is unknown owing to the lack of long-term follow-up. Haematometra may result from either cervical stenosis or the formation of loculated areas within the uterine cavity subsequent to the development of uterine synechiae. Simple cervical dilatation and drainage may well be all that is required, but some cases may warrant repeat TCRE or even hysterectomy.

The development of cyclical lower abdominal pain after TCRE has been reported, probably resulting from small islands of endometrium becoming buried in the myometrium. Where analgesics do not suffice, hysterectomy should be seriously considered.

Pregnancy

Pregnancy after TCRE, resulting in a favourable outcome (Kilby *et al*, 1994), has been reported. Sterilisation may therefore be performed at the time of TCRE on those patients who have no desire to retain their fertility.

Outcome

DeCherney *et al* (1987) reported amenorrhoea in 95% (20/21) of patients with intractable uterine bleeding after TCRE. No published report since has equalled their achievement. More recent studies have achieved amenorrhoea in 22–42% of patients, depending on the length of follow-up and definition of amenorrhoea (Magos *et al*, 1991; Cooper *et al*, 1992; Pinion *et al*, 1994), with better results being achieved in patients over 35 years of age (Magos *et al*, 1991). Local experience has shown 32% (29/91) of patients to be amenorrhoeic after TCRE with a minimum of 3-year follow-up.

Dysmenorrhoea improves in approximately 65% of patients, as may premenstual symptoms of breast tenderness, bloating and mood swings (Dwyer *et al*, 1993). An identical improvement rate was also recorded in our series (59/91).

Patient satisfaction surveys conducted between 4 months and 3 years after TCRE report satisfaction rates between 70% and 85%, and up to 95% if a repeat procedure is performed on the 5–20% of patients who were initially dissatisfied (Magos *et al*, 1991; Rankin and Steinberg, 1992; Dwyer *et al*, 1993; Pinion *et al*, 1994). In our patient satisfaction survey of 91 patients with a minimum of 3-year follow-up, 81% of patients had an improvement in their menstrual symptoms and 66% were satisfied; 19% experienced no benefit and expressed a wish to have a hysterectomy. However, trend analysis in gynaecological surgery shows a reduced need for hysterectomy over a 5-year period (Table 3). Our analysis demonstrates that endometrial resection avoids the need for hysterectomy in a significant proportion of patients.

In order to obtain a better understanding of TCRE using patient feedback 273 consecutive patients treated between 1989 and 1994 were asked to complete a self- administered annual questionnaire. This asked details of patient opinion, choice and satisfaction with treatment, further surgery required as well as standard parameters of symptom improvement (Figures 2, 3, 4). Of the 273 patients, 91% responded at year 1 and 73% by year 4. Approximately 67% remained satisfied throughout years 1 to 4 of follow-up. Accumulative re-operation may increase with time from 13% in year 1 to 24% by the end of year 4. The procedure achieved a 30% amenorrhoea rate and a further 41% of patients had lighter periods. Following database interrogation, satisfaction with the outcome was most likely:

1. In women with regular menstrual cycles (Figure 4).
2. In women over 45 years of age (Figure 2).
3. When the procedure was performed during the proliferative phase (Figure 3).

Table 3. Hysterectomy and transcervical resection of the endometrium (TCRE), Liverpool Women's Hospital 1989–93*

Year	Number of hysterectomies	Number of TCREs	Number of major cases on waiting list at end of year
1989	97	0	152
1990	109	8	188
1991	99	46	169
1992	79	104	88
1993	62	59	60

95% confidence intervals: 1991=2.85–4.95; 1992=8.01–40.18; 1993=5.82–28.90
*From Armatage *et al* (1995)

Key points

- Transcervical resection of the endometrium (TCRE) is a successful treatment for menorrhagia.
- Preparation of the endometrium is not required before surgery.
- Appropriate training is essential.
- TCRE is not a sterilisation procedure.

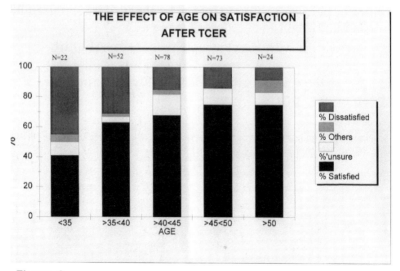

Figure. 2

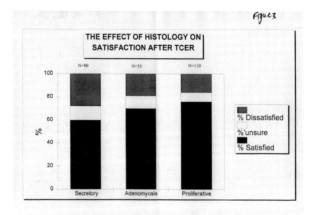

Figure. 3

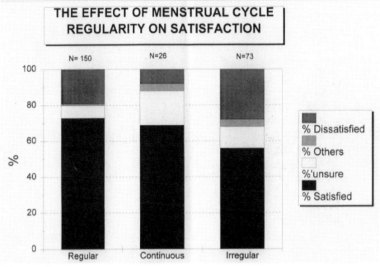

Figure. 4

References

Armatage RJ, Quenby S, Granger K, Faquharson RG (1995) Trends in gynaecological surgery. *Lancet* **845**: 129

Cooper MJW, Magos A, Baumann R, Rees MCP (1992) The effect of endometrial resection on menstrual blood loss. *Gynaecol Endosc* **1**: 195–8

DeCherney AH, Polan ML (1983) Hysteroscopic resection of intrauterine lesions and intractable bleeding. *Obstet Gynecol* **61**: 392–7

DeCherney AH, Diamond MP, Lavy G, Polan ML (1987) Endometrial ablation for intractable uterine bleeding: hysteroscopic resection. *Obstet Gynecol* **70**: 668–9

Dwyer N, Hutton J, Stirrat GM (1993) Randomised controlled trial comparing endometrial resection with abdominal hysterectomy for the treatment of menorrhagia. *Br J Obstet Gynaecol* **100**: 237–43

Ewen SP, Manners B, Sutton GJC (1994) A randomised study to compare the effects of Zoladex and danazol on endometrial atrophy prior to endometrial resection. *Gynaecol Endosc* **3** (Suppl 1): 28

Hospital Inpatient Enquiry (1985) HMSO/OPCS, London: 1

Kilby M, Clubb AW, O'Brien PMS (1994) Pregnancy following endometrial resection. *J Obstet Gynaecol* **14**: 17–18

MacDonald R, Tiernan C, Singer A (1994) Endometrial resection: does pre-operative Zoladex influence outcome? *Gynaecol Endosc* 3 (Suppl 1): 29–30

Magos AL, Baumann R, Turnbull AC (1989) Transcervical resection of the endometrium in women with menorrhagia. *Br Med J* **298**: 1209–12

Magos AL, Baumann R, Lockwood GM, Turnbull AC (1991) Experience with the first 250 endometrial resections for menorrhagia. *Lancet* **337**: 1074–8

Morbidity Statistics from General Practice 1981–1982 (1986) HMSO, London

Neuwirth RS, Amin JH (1976) Excision of submucous fibroids with hysteroscopic control. *Am J Obstet Gynecol* **126**: 95–9

Pantaleoni DC (1869) On endoscopic examination of the cavity of the womb. *Medical Press Circular* **8**: 26–7

Pinion SB, Parkin DE, Abramovich DR *et al* (1994) Randomised trial of hysterectomy, endometrial laser, ablation, and transcervical endometrial resection for dysfunctional uterine bleeding. *Br Med J* **309**: 979–83

Pyper RJD, Haeri AD (1991) A review of 80 endometrial resections for menorrhagia. *Br J Obstet Gynaecol* **98**: 1049–54

Rankin L, Steinberg LH (1992) Transcervical resection of the endometrium: a review of 400 consecutive patients. *Br J Obstet Gynaecol* **99**: 911–4

van Herendael B (1993) Hazards and dangers of operative hysteroscopy. In: Sutton C, Diamond M, eds. *Endoscopic Surgery for Gynaecologists*. WB Saunders, London: 355–61

11 An introduction to the principles and safety of electrosurgery

S Veck

With the advent of minimal access surgery, the use of different energy sources has made a tremendous contribution to the treatment of modalities in many gynaecological disorders. The trainee must be clear in the understanding of not only the application of energy sources, but also the principles behind their use. This chapter has thus been written to provide insight into avoiding patient injury as well as safety of use.

High frequency (HF) electrosurgery has been used in surgical practice for approximately 70 years. The first devices used a spark gap generator to provide coagulation, and a valve oscillator for cutting. The next generation used valve generators, offering much improved control of setting for cutting and coagulation current. During the early 1970s, modern transistor technology further advanced the realisation of numerous application possibilities. Many of these devices are still used today.

Some would recognise that surgery has taken a quantum leap during the last decade and, as such, has imposed more specific demands on an electrosurgical generator. Much of this expanded demand has been due to advances in surgery, endoscopy, and especially the introduction of minimal access surgery (MAS). With the use of modern microprocessor technology, the surgeon can utilise the full advantages that these systems may offer with increased levels of safety.

Electrosurgical generators provide usually four modalities, cutting, blended cut, coagulation and bipolar coagulation. Many generators today offer specialised

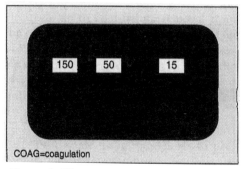

COAG=coagulation

Figure 1. Diagram of an electrosurgical generator

coagulation, eg. argon enhanced plasma coagulation and bipolar cutting (Figure 1).

Physical principles of HF electrosurgery

To eliminate muscle and nerve stimulation, the incoming electrical frequency of 50 Hz is transformed to between 300 kHz and 1mHz. It is essential to understand that electrosurgery operates on a simple circuit system. The cutting or coagulation current flows from the electrosurgical generator through an active cable and instrument, usually forceps or a hand-held pencil. The desired current then flows through the patient, taking the pathway of least resistance, and is removed by means of a conductive return plate which returns to the generator. As the patient is acting as the major pathway for this current, it is vital that all safety measures are taken to prevent inadvertent burns. It is possible to burn a patient from either the active or return point. The intended active point is usually very small, eg. forceps tips or needle/blade electrode, producing high current concentration in order to provide a cutting or coagulation effect.

Return plates are designed to be highly conductive to remove current safely, however, if this surface area is reduced because of poor contact of the tissue, or is sited on poor conductive tissue, the current can concentrate, and in certain conditions a burn may occur. It is clear that the function of a return plate is vital in preventing injury. The plate should be sited in a well vascularised area, such as the upper arm or thigh, and never over bony prominences or scar tissue. Additionally, any hair or dry, flaky skin should be removed to ensure good contact of the plate. Some manufacturers of electrosurgical generators have developed split plates, which have a feedback to the generator, providing contact quality and quantity information. Should the status of the plate be compromised, an audible alarm and immediate shutdown of power occurs.

As previously mentioned, modern electrosurgical generators can provide numerous modalities; cutting is achieved by using a small electrode, eg. needle/blade electrode, with the voltage above 200 vp (volts peak) to develop a spark and a continuous sinusoid waveform (Figure 2). The spark jumps from the electrode to the tissue, rapidly heating the cells in the tissue so that the fluid in the cells vapourises causing the cell to rupture. The rupturing cells form the incision in the path of the electrode, severing tissue as cleanly as a scalpel. Cutting may therefore be described as the electromechanical disruption of tissue, resulting from the passage of high radio frequency currents through that tissue. Where potential for bleeding is possible, a blended cut is available, ie. cutting with intermittent coagulation (Figure 3). This is achieved by modulating the cut waveform; in most generators various degrees of blend can be selected to obtain the desired effect.

Types of coagulation

Monopolar

There are three types of coagulation modes, each mode having a beneficial function on certain types of tissue. Spray coagulation provides a relatively superficial form of coagulation, employing relatively high voltages. The instrument tip is held close to the tissue but never comes into contact with it. The spray coagulation effect is specific for underwater surgery or in areas of diffused haemorrhage. Fulguration is also a high voltage mode of coagulation

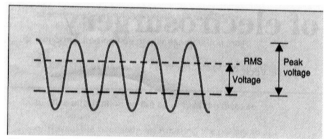

Figure 2. Cut waveform

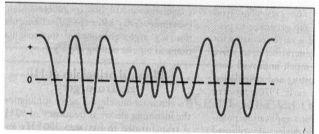

Figure 3. Blended cut waveform

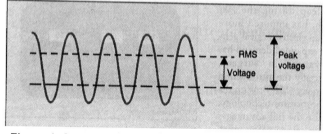

Figure 4. Coagulation waveform

(Figure 4) which provides a substantial depth of coagulation to major bleeds. Dessication, the most frequently used technique, is the slow drying out of tissues; when the electrode is in contact with tissue, very little, if any, sparking should occur. Spray, however, appears the most powerful of all modes of coagulation, because of the high voltage and intense rapid sparking.

Bipolar

Bipolar coagulation and cutting have both the active and return electrodes incorporated into the instrument. The current typically flows down the active portion, through the tissue to be cut or coagulated, and is returned via the return portion of the instrument, therefore no current flows through the patient's body. Recent developments in bipolar technology have produced instruments for MAS, providing increased levels of safety.

MAS

MAS has without doubt produced an alternative facet of surgery. The use of electrosurgery in gynaecological MAS is well documented, although it lost favour as a surgical modality because of damage caused to adjacent organs and structures. With the continuing development of electro-surgical technology, however, many safer options are now available. In particular, bipolar cutting and coagulation, as previously mentioned, has generated renewed interest in this type of tissue management.

Risks

There are unfortunately increased levels of risk when using electrosurgery in MAS. This is partly owing to the areas that are out of direct view of the surgeon. There are four main safety concerns when using monopolar current:

- capacitive coupling
- direct coupling
- insulation failure
- thermal injury.

All these areas of risk can be reduced with care and attention. A good image of the operative site is paramount, as well as adequate provision for irrigation and aspiration of fluids and smoke particulates. The Trendelenberg position is useful when ensuring that other tissues, such as bowel tissue, do not form part of the operative site. Capacitive coupling can occur when mixing plastic and metal cannulae, an example of this is when a plastic gripper is placed over a metal cannula. This can effectively insulate any capacitive charge from dissipating through the abdominal wall. Under certain circumstances, eg. when using high voltage current, a discharge of this capacitive current could contact tissue in close proximity to the cannula, such as the bowel. This could then result in a burn, without the surgeon being aware, because it is out of direct view.

Direct coupling occurs when instruments are crossed, or come into direct contact. An example of this is when the monopolar hook electrode touches the laparoscope, which gives rise to a burn to any tissue adjacent to the laparoscope. Spatial orientation is therefore vital.

Insulation of instruments and cables is a high priority; any break in insulation can cause inadvertent burns. If the break is small, high current concentration can develop, producing a surgical effect in an otherwise unintended site (Figure 5). An indication of this could be the lack of any surgical effect at the operative site and the presumption that a higher power setting is required.

Thermal injury can be avoided simply by ensuring that after using a monopolar instrument, sufficient time is given for the electrode tip to cool before removal from the operation site. Electrode tips can retain heat for several seconds after use, so it is also good practice when withdrawing the instrument to do so under direct vision until it is out of the body cavity.

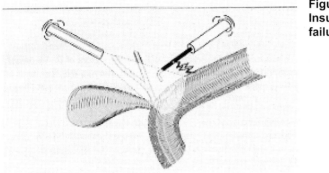

**Figure 5.
Insulation
failure**

Guidelines for use

Listed are some useful guidelines to prevent patient and user injury:

- always check the integrity of insulation, of cables and instruments before use
- use the bipolar technique if possible
- pass the laparoscope through all metal, or all plastic cannulae/anchor sets
- use the lowest power setting practical
- be aware of the effects of capacitance, direct coupling and residual heat
- use low-voltage coagulation
- don't use a plastic anchor (gripper) with a metal cannula
- don't activate the electrode unless it is clearly in view and in direct contact with tissue
- don't use insertion ports with sharp edges
- don't re-use single use electrodes
- don't use high-voltage spray coagulation
- don't leave the electrode lying on the patient between uses, but place in a holster.

Conclusion

Electrosurgery can offer a wide range of applications and remains an integral part of the surgical equipment, partly owing to the increased levels of safety now available in the electrosurgical tools. It is imperative, however, that adequate training is given at all levels to ensure an optimum safe environment.

Key points

- Become familiar with the functions and limitations of your electrosurgical generator.
- Be aware of the generator patient plate alarm system.
- Ensure that both the quality and quantity, as well as the position of the plate is good.
- Always use the lowest power setting practical to achieve the desired surgical effect.
- To prevent inadvertent burns to both patients and surgeon, check integrity of insulation to all instruments and cables before use.
- If a product is single use, it should be discarded, as re-use could result in insulation failure or in the case of plates, reduced contact quality.
- Regular service checks are important to ensure safety of the electrosurgical generator.

12 Obstetric thromboprophylaxis

C Nelson-Piercy

Thromboembolism in pregnancy is a major cause of maternal mortality. Pregnancy, particularly caesarean section, increases the risk of thrombosis. This chapter discusses the risk factors, the drugs used and the indications for prophylaxis of thromboembolism in pregnancy.

Pulmonary embolism (PE) in pregnancy and the puerperium kills about ten women each year in the UK, and accounts for one in five of all direct maternal deaths. Thromboembolism has been a leading cause of maternal mortality in the UK since the Confidential Enquiries into Maternal Deaths began in 1973 (Department of Health, Welsh Office, Scottish Home and Health Department and Department of Health and Social Services, Northern Ireland, 1994). Pregnancy increases the risk of thromboembolism sixfold (Royal College of General Practitioners, 1967) and caesarean section further increases this risk approximately tenfold. Exact figures for the incidence of non-fatal PE and deep vein thrombosis (DVT) are not available, although it is probably in the region of 0.5%–1% in developed countries.

Risk factors

The hypercoagulable state of pregnancy results from an alteration in the balance of clotting factors and endogenous anticoagulants in favour of blood clotting. These physiological haemostatic adaptations to pregnancy act to create a relatively thrombogenic state from early pregnancy. These are factors, along with the venous stasis associated with pressure of the gravid uterus on the inferior vena cava, which are present in all pregnant women. Specific factors, such as increased maternal age, increased parity, obesity and operative delivery, will further increase the risk. Other important risk factors include previous thromboembolism and thrombophilia (Table 1). These are discussed below.

Drugs used for thromboprophylaxis

Warfarin

Warfarin crosses the placenta, is teratogenic, and must therefore be avoided during the first trimester. The teratogenic risk usually quoted (limited to chondrodysplasia punctata) is about 5%, but this is probably an overestimate. Furthermore, the period of risk is between the sixth and twelfth week of gestation, so conception on warfarin therapy is not dangerous, provided that the warfarin is replaced by heparin within 2 weeks of the first missed period.

Warfarin's association with microcephaly and neuro-logical abnormalities when used in the second trimester is almost certainly related to over-anticoagulation of the mother and therefore the fetus. There is a significant risk of both maternal (retroplacental) and fetal (intracerebral) bleeding when warfarin is used in the third trimester, and particularly after 36 weeks. Although some units do use warfarin for obstetric thromboprophylaxis in the second and early third trimester, this should only be under close supervision.

Table 1. Factors contributing to the increased risk of thromboembolism in pregnancy and the puerperium

Changes common to all pregnant women	Haemostatic factors	Increased levels of blood clotting factors, particularly fibrinogen
		Decreased fibrinolysis
		Decreased levels of endogenous anticoagulants, eg. antithrombin III, protein S
		Venous stasis
Additional risk factors	Obesity	
	Increased maternal age	
	Increased maternal parity	
	Operative delivery	
	Thrombophilia	
	Previous thromboembolism	
	Prolonged bed rest	
	Pre-eclampsia	

The single undisputed indication for warfarin use in pregnancy is for thromboprophylaxis in women with metal prosthetic heart valve replacements, in whom the risk of thrombosis is high and for whom thrombosis carries a high mortality. These women require full anticoagulation throughout pregnancy.

Heparin

Subcutaneous heparin, which does not cross the placenta and therefore has no adverse effects on the fetus, is the most commonly used mode of thromboprophylaxis in pregnancy in the UK (Greer and de Swiet, 1993).

The risk of heparin-induced osteoporosis is particularly pertinent in obstetrics, first because heparin use may be for up to 10 months, and second because pregnancy and breast-feeding themselves cause reversible bone demineralisation. There have been several reports of vertebral collapse associated with heparin use in pregnancy (de Swiet, 1995). The incidence of symptomatic osteoporosis associated with heparin use in pregnancy may be as high as 2% (Dahlman, 1993) and it is this risk which must be balanced against the risk of recurrent thromboembolism. Heparin-induced osteopenia may be subclinical, and studies have shown that thromboprophylaxis with heparin in pregnancy may cause a 5% reduction in bone density, equivalent to 2 years postmenopausal bone loss. Fortunately, however, bone density is seen to improve once heparin therapy is discontinued postpartum.

Thrombocytopenia is another rare but potentially dangerous side-effect of heparin treatment. There are two forms of heparin-induced thrombocytopenia: the first is an immediate-onset, non-idiosyncratic reaction which is of little clinical importance; the second is a later (6–10 days), idiosyncratic, immune-mediated form which is more serious and is associated with paradoxical thrombosis. There are reports of heparin-induced thrombocytopenia in pregnancy, but in the UK this complication of heparin therapy is unusual.

Low molecular weight heparins

Low molecular weight heparins (LMWHs), produced by enzymatic or chemical breakdown of the heparin molecule, may offer advantages over standard, unfractionated heparin (UH). The most obvious of these in obstetrics, where the timescale of prophylaxis is much longer than in surgery, is the increased bioavailability and longer half-life of LMWHs, which together allow for once-daily administration.

Because LMWHs are composed of shorter molecules than UH, the ratio of anti-Xa (antithrombotic) to anti-IIa (anticoagulant) activity, which is inversely proportional to the molecular weight, is increased. This property has led to claims of an improved clinical benefit (antithrombosis) to risk (inadvertent anticoagulation and bleeding) ratio. LMWHs have less effect on platelet aggregation and less inhibition of platelet function than UH, which reduce the risk of early thrombocytopenia. LMWHs are less capable than UH of activating resting platelets to release platelet factor 4, and they bind less well to platelet factor 4, thereby decreasing the risk of late-onset immune thrombocytopenia.

LMWHs have been studied extensively outside pregnancy. They are certainly as effective and may well be safer than UH. They are gaining popularity for obstetric thromboprophylaxis, largely because of their convenience and acceptability (Nelson-Piercy, 1994). It is hoped that they may also be associated with a lower risk of osteoporosis, although this has yet to be demonstrated and is currently under study (Shefras and Farquharson, 1994).

The increased circulating blood volume in pregnancy necessitates a higher dose of heparin (10 000 units, twice daily) and LMWH (eg. enoxaparin, 40 mg daily; dalteparin, 5000 units daily) than is recommended outside pregnancy. Heparin is usually given as self-administered subcutaneous injections.

Aspirin

Antiplatelet therapy has been shown to be effective in reducing the risk of venous thrombosis in surgical and medical patients. The use of aspirin for thromboprophylaxis in pregnancy has never been submitted to randomised, controlled trial. It is known from the results of the Collaborative Low-Dose

Aspirin Study in Pregnancy (CLASP) that low-dose aspirin is safe in pregnancy. It does not seem unreasonable, therefore, to use aspirin in situations where the risk of thrombosis is not deemed sufficiently high to warrant subcutaneous heparin.

Indications for thromboprophylaxis

Since thromboprophylaxis with heparin or warfarin is not without risk, as described above, a policy of universal thromboprophylaxis is not appropriate, and some assessment of individual risk is needed before deciding whether and for how long thromboprophylaxis is needed (Table 2).

Previous thromboembolism

When assessing the need for thromboprophylaxis in pregnancy, an accurate history of previous thromboembolic events is vital. The clinical features of both DVT and PE are not specific and, if used alone, are notoriously unreliable; the diagnosis will be wrong in up to 50% of cases. This is further compounded in pregnancy because leg oedema (which may often be asymmetrical) is common. Further, up to 75% of women experience breathlessness at some stage in pregnancy. Thus, it is important to establish an objective diagnosis of thromboembolism in pregnancy, and similarly to enquire whether a diagnosis of previous thromboembolism was objectively confirmed.

Opinion varies concerning the level of prophylaxis for women with a single previous thromboembolic event. Because of the risks, particularly of osteoporosis, we reserve antenatal heparin prophylaxis for women with thrombophilia, thromboembolism in the current pregnancy, a history of recurrent thromboembolic events, and those with a family history of thromboembolism. Women with a single previous thromboembolic event, but without any of the above features, receive heparin prophylaxis in labour and the puerperium and low-dose aspirin (75 mg daily) antenatally.

Table 2. Protocol for obstetric thromboprophylaxis			
Risk category	**Risk factors**		**Prophylaxis**
High risk	Thrombophilia		Antenatal: subcutaneous heparin or LMWH
	Previous thromboembolism and antiphospholipid syndrome		Intrapartum: subcutaneous heparin or LMWH
	Previous thromboembolism and family history of thromboembolism		Postpartum: subcutaneous heparin or LMWH for 3–7 days followed by subcutaneous heparin or LMWH or warfarin for a total of 6 weeks
	Recurrent thromboembolism		
	Thromboembolism in current pregnancy		
Low risk	One previous thromboembolic episode (without a family history of thromboembolism)		Antenatal: low-dose (75 mg) aspirin
			Intrapartum: subcutaneous heparin or LMWH
			Postpartum: as above
Additional risk	Two or more of:	Caesarean section	Intrapartum: subcutaneous heparin or LMWH
		Obesity (>96 kg)	Postpartum: subcutaneous heparin or LMWH for 3–4 days
		Age >35 years	
LMWH=low molecular weight heparin			

Thrombophilia

Women with thrombophilia are at a high risk of recurrent thromboembolic events in pregnancy and the puerperium. Thrombophilia may be divided into inherited and acquired forms (Table 3). A history of recurrent, atypical (eg. axillary vein) or unprovoked (not associated with combined oral contraceptive, pregnancy, trauma or surgery) thromboembolism should stimulate a search for thrombophilia. Similarly, a family history of thromboembolism is important, since it may indicate inherited thrombophilia. A full thrombophilia screen should be performed. A simple 'clotting screen' is unhelpful, although prolonged activated partial thromboplastin time (APTT) may suggest lupus anticoagulant.

Table 3. Types of thrombophilia	
Inherited thrombophilia	Protein C
	Protein S
	Antithrombin III
	Activated protein C resistance
Acquired thrombophilia	Lupus anticoagulant
	Anticardiolipin antibodies

Protein C deficiency, protein S deficiency and antithrombin III deficiency are all rare, but the recently discovered activated protein C resistance (APCR) is 5–10 times more common than any of the other known deficiencies of anticoagulant proteins. APCR is caused by a defective factor V caused by a single missense mutation in the factor V gene (the Leiden mutation). Hellgren *et al* (1995) demonstrated a prevalence of APCR of almost 60% in women with thromboembolic complications during pregnancy, and in 30% of women with thromboembolic complications during treatment with oral contraceptives. Since this defect is relatively common in the general population, the authors of the above study suggest that it may be reasonable to perform a general screening for APCR during early pregnancy or before prescription of oral contraceptives. Certainly there is now a case for screening anyone who has had a previous history of thromboembolism.

Women with antiphospholipid antibodies (lupus anticoagulant or anticardiolipin antibodies) receive low-dose aspirin antenatally for fetal reasons. If they have had a previous thromboembolic event or late pregnancy loss they are classified as 'high risk' and receive antenatal subcutaneous heparin prophylaxis. The risk of recurrent thrombosis in antiphospholipid syndrome may be as high as 70%, and some women will be on long-term warfarin treatment outside pregnancy.

Additional risk factors

The Royal College of Obstetricians and Gynaecologists (RCOG) has recently published recommendations for prophylaxis in obstetrics (RCOG, 1995). These include a risk assessment profile for thromboembolism in caesarean section. Risk factors include age >35 years, obesity >80 kg, parity >four, gross varicose veins, pre-eclampsia and immobility >4 days before surgery. However, prophylaxis to cover delivery should not be limited to those undergoing caesarean section, since some women who die of PE following childbirth have had vaginal deliveries. At Queen Charlotte's Hospital, we recommend prophylaxis for obese women over the age of 37 years, even for a normal delivery. The time of greatest risk for thrombosis is probably around the time of delivery and the early puerperium. Therefore women who qualify for intrapartum heparin prophylaxis can probably safely discontinue this after 3–4 days.

Antenatal management

Having decided into which risk category a woman falls, she should then be counselled appropriately. This is particularly so for high-risk women, considering the relative risks of heparin-induced osteoporosis and recurrent thromboembolism.

When monitoring women receiving long-term heparin:

- A platelet count should be performed in all patients on heparin therapy to check for heparin-induced thrombocytopenia. Since immune/late heparin-induced thrombocytopenia occurs after 6 days of treatment, a platelet count is performed 1 week after starting heparin treatment, and then approximately monthly.

- A coagulation screen is required (approximately monthly) to ensure that the patient is not receiving anticoagulant doses of heparin. It should remain normal (not prolonged for more than 2–3 seconds beyond control).

- Heparin levels, based on anti-Xa assays, can be monitored and should not exceed 0.2 units/ml.

- The assay must be calibrated for the particular UH or LMWH in use. Monitoring with a coagulation screen alone is acceptable where anti-Xa assays are not available.

Sadly, there is no way to predict which women will develop heparin-induced osteoporosis. The serum calcium level gives no indication of the bone stores of calcium.

Intrapartum management

Because of the high risk of thromboembolism immediately postpartum, heparin should not be discontinued during labour. For those 'low-risk' women starting prophylaxis with heparin intrapartum, the first dose should ideally be administered before delivery. Heparin in low/prophylactic doses does not interfere with the activation of normal haemostatic mechanisms at the site of injury, but only lowers the risk of in-situ, spontaneous clot formation. A coagulation screen should be checked before the siting of an epidural/spinal block. A normal clotting time (not prolonged for more than 2–3 seconds) indicates no extra risk of epidural haematoma. In controlled studies, at least 10 000 patients have been given the combination of LMWH in prophylactic doses and epidural/spinal anaesthesia without complications. If appropriate, the heparin injection can be delayed until after the epidural has been sited.

Postpartum management

Neither warfarin or heparin are excreted in breast milk, thus breast-feeding is not contraindicated with their use. The important principle is that prophylaxis with either warfarin or subcutaneous heparin be continued for 6 weeks after delivery. The advantages of changing to warfarin within the first week after delivery are that exposure to heparin is minimised and there is no further need for self-administered, subcutaneous injections. The disadvantage relates to the need for closer monitoring and venepuncture. Women who have received more than 10–12 weeks' heparin therapy should be offered postpartum bone densitometry. This is usually done by means of a dual X-ray absorptiometry (DEXA) scan, which compares the bone density of the spine and hip to the mean for age- and sex- matched, non-pregnant controls.

Key points

- Pregnancy increases the risk of thromboembolism, and pulmonary embolism remains a leading cause of maternal mortality.

- Women at high risk of recurrent thrombosis should receive antenatal, intrapartum and postnatal thromboprophylaxis.
- Caesarean section further increases the risk of thromboembolism, and thromboprophylaxis should be offered to any woman with additional risk factors.

References

Dahlman TC (1993) Osteoporotic fractures and the recurrence of thrombo-embolism during pregnancy and the puerperium in 184 women undergoing thromboprophylaxis with heparin. *Am J Obstet Gynecol* **168**: 1265–70

Department of Health, Welsh Office, Scottish Home and Health Department and Department of Health and Social Services, Northern Ireland (1994) *Confidential Enquiries into Maternal Deaths in the United Kingdom 1988–90.* HMSO, London

de Swiet M (1995) Thrombo-embolism. In: de Swiet M, ed. *Medical Disorders in Obstetric Practice*. 3rd edn. Blackwell Science, Oxford

Greer IA, de Swiet M (1993) Thrombosis prophylaxis in obstetrics and gynaecology. *Br J Obstet Gynaecol* **100**: 37–40

Hellgren M, Svensson PJ, Dahlback B (1995) Resistance to activated protein C as a basis for venous thromboembolism associated with pregnancy and oral contraceptives. *Am J Obstet Gynecol* **173**: 210–13

Nelson-Piercy C (1994) Low molecular weight heparin for obstetric thromboprophylaxis. *Br J Obstet Gynaecol* **101**: 6–8

Royal College of General Practitioners (1967) Oral contraception and thrombo-embolic disease. *J R Coll Gen Pract* **13**: 267–9

Royal College of Obstetricians and Gynaecologists (1995) *Thrombo-embolic Disease in Gynaecology and Pregnancy: Recommendations for Prophylaxis*. RCOG, London

Shefras J, Farquharson RG (1994) Bone Density Studies in pregnant women receiving heparin. *Eur J Obs Gyn* **52**: 171–175

13 The pelvic floor sequelae of childbirth

AH Sultan, AK Monga, SL Stanton

For centuries the structure and function of the pelvic floor and anal sphincter have remained enigmatic. Great strides made in new imaging techniques over the last decade has enabled a better understanding of this complex and dynamic structure. We can now explore pelvic floor dysfunction.

MacArthur *et al* (1991) stated that:

> '*Childbirth must be far and away the major cause of chronic health problems among women in the child rearing years.*'

This concluding remark follows analysis of 11701 postal questionnaires completed 1–9 years after delivery. A total of 47% of women reported at least one new symptom within 3 months of delivery such as backache, headache, haemorrhoids, depression, and bowel and bladder symptoms, persisting for a minimum of 6 weeks. Glazener *et al* (1995) analysed the postnatal maternal morbidity in a random sample of 1249 deliveries. They found that 76% reported at least one health problem 8 weeks after delivery. Women were particularly prone to problems after assisted vaginal delivery.

Urinary incontinence, anal incontinence and uterovaginal prolapse are the major pelvic floor sequelae of vaginal delivery. These symptoms may present late in life, and as female life expectancy in the Western World has doubled to 80 years in the last century, increasing numbers of women are being affected. To maintain a better quality of life attempts are being made to reduce pelvic floor and perineal trauma during childbirth. This trauma may result in connective tissue damage, neuropathy and muscle injury which are thought to be the three main contributory factors to the development of incontinence and prolapse.

Urinary incontinence

Although involuntary loss of urine is reported by about 20% of women 3 months after delivery (Sleep, 1991), the community prevalence of urinary incontinence appears to be underestimated. In one study (Thomas *et al*, 1984), conducted in the Brent and Harrow health district in London, the prevalence of urinary incontinence known to Health and Social Services was 0.2% in the age group 15–64 years and 2.5% in those greater than 65 years, but when a postal survey was conducted in the same area it was found to be 8.5% and 11.6% respectively. It is believed that for every case of recognised incontinence there are at least 20 unrecognised cases.

Although vaginal delivery is implicated as a major aetiological factor in urinary incontinence the exact mechanism is unclear. Using different diagnostic techniques, pelvic and pudendal neuropathy has been demonstrated in women with urinary stress incontinence (Anderson, 1984; Gilpin *et al*, 1989; Smith *et al*, 1989). While delayed pudendal nerve conduction has been shown to recover (Snooks *et al*, 1984; Sultan *et al*, 1994a), neuropathy has also been shown to progressively deteriorate after the first vaginal delivery. This appears to be related to ageing rather than subsequent delivery (Snooks *et al*, 1990; Mallett *et al*, 1994).

Barnick and Cardozo (1993), using concentric needle electromyography (EMG) of the urethral sphincter, found no correlation between denervation/reinnervation changes and genuine stress incontinence, and demonstrated that these changes were associated with improved urethral function. In contrast to other studies they concluded that denervation is not a major aetiological factor in the development of genuine stress incontinence.

More recently, eight women with stress incontinence and ten nulliparous controls were examined using EMG recordings of the right and left pubococcygeus muscle via wire electrodes (Deindl *et al*, 1994). They found that childbirth induced both qualitative and quantitative changes in the pelvic floor contributing to the development of stress incontinence. Their findings suggested that sphincter weakness resulted not only from loss of individual motor units but also from altered behaviour of the remaining units, such that there was asynchronous activity between the two sides of the pubococcygeus muscle. In other words, during straining or urination, when the levators should be relaxed, inappropriate muscle activity was detected on one side; during a voluntary contraction there was inappropriate inhibition of firing units on the contralateral side.

Mechanical trauma to the urethropelvic ligaments, the supporting structures of the urethra, has been reported in stress incontinent women (Klutke *et al*, 1990). Another magnetic resonance imaging study could not substantiate this finding and denied the existence of the urethropelvic ligaments. However, degeneration of the levator ani muscle was observed in 45% of women with stress incontinence (Kirschner-Hermanns *et al*, 1993).

The exact aetiological mechanism is unknown but is probably multifactorial. Although vaginal delivery undoubtedly remains a major aetiological factor (Sleep, 1991; Glazener *et al*, 1995), some women appear to be at greater risk of developing symptoms; this may be related to abnormal connective tissue (Keane *et al*, 1992).

Genital prolapse

Genital prolapse is a consequence of failure of the fibromuscular supports that confine the pelvic organs within the pelvic cavity. Fifty per cent of parous women have some degree of genital prolapse but only 10–20% are symptomatic and severity increases with age. Two per cent of symptomatic prolapse occurs in nulliparous women (Nichols and Randall, 1983) implying that there may be a congenital weakness of connective tissue. In addition, genital prolapse is rare in black women, suggesting that genetic differences exist.

The connective tissue of the pelvic floor is vital for support of the pelvic structures, and is influenced by pregnancy, childbirth and ageing. Whether congenital or acquired, connective tissue defects appear to be important in the aetiology of prolapse and urinary stress incontinence. Patients with genital prolapse exhibit increased striae and joint hypermobility (Norton *et al*, 1992), features which are present in patients with other connective tissue disorders, namely Ehlers-Danlos syndrome and Marfan's syndrome. Women with Ehlers-Danlos syndrome have increased complaints of incontinence and prolapse (McIntosh *et al*, 1993). A 40% decrease in skin total collagen content is reported in women with genuine stress incontinence compared to continent controls (Ulmsten *et al*, 1987). A significant reduction in type I:III collagen ratios is reported in women with genital prolapse and nulliparous women with genuine stress incontinence. There is now evidence to suggest that women with genital prolapse have reduced total collagen content and an increase in immature cross linkage (Jackson *et al*, 1995).

The single major factor leading to the development of genital prolapse appears to be vaginal delivery (Parks *et al*, 1977; Snooks *et al*, 1984, 1990; Gilpin *et al*, 1989). Histological, histochemical and electromyographic studies of the pubococcygeus muscle and pubocervical fascia have shown evidence of greater denervation in women with prolapse compared to those without, and this occurs as a result of vaginal delivery (Gilpin *et al*, 1989; Smith *et al*, 1989). Greater parity is associated with increasing prolapse. The World Health Organisation population report (1984) suggested that prolapse was up to seven times more common in women who had more than seven children compared to those with one. Prolapse occurring during pregnancy is rare but is thought to be mediated by the effects of progesterone and relaxin. In addition, the increase in intra-abdominal pressure puts added strain on the pelvic floor and a raised intra-abdominal pressure outside of pregnancy (eg. chronic cough or constipation) is also a risk (Spence-Jones *et al*, 1994).

The process of ageing can result in loss of collagen and weakness of fascia as well as a progression in neuropathy (Laurberg and Swash, 1989). Brincat *et al* (1983) demonstrated the beneficial effect of oestrogen on collagen crosslinkages in skin. As oestrogen receptors have been identified in the levator ani and anal sphincter muscle, postmenopausal oestrogen deficiency may predispose to pelvic floor weakness (Haadem *et al*, 1991).

Mechanical displacement as a result of gynaecological surgery, such as colposuspension, may lead to the development of a rectocele or enterocoele (Wiskind *et al*, 1992). Whether this occurs in patients with an inherent predisposition requires further evaluation.

The mechanism behind the development of genital prolapse, however, remains unresolved. While denervation of the pelvic floor has long been linked to the development of genital prolapse, there has been a rekindling of the concept of support defects originally suggested by White in 1912. This has led to the development of techniques specifically directed at repair of these anatomic defects (Shull *et al*, 1994).

Anal incontinence

The understanding of the pathogenesis of anal incontinence has evolved along very similar lines to that of urinary incontinence and genital prolapse. Parks (1975) postulated that excessive straining, particularly with constipation or prolonged pushing during childbirth, leads to traction injury of the pelvic and pudendal nerves. This neuropathy leads to atrophy and weakness of the pelvic floor anal sphincter complex.

Two prospective studies (Snooks *et al*, 1984; Allen *et al*, 1990) have demonstrated that a denervation process is initiated during vaginal delivery. Allen *et al* found that 80% of primiparae showed evidence of reinnervation following denervation. They suggested that denervation is the first step in a pathway ultimately leading to incontinence. Short-term prospective studies have not demonstrated a relationship between abnormal neurophysiological tests and symptoms of anal incontinence (Snooks *et al*, 1984; Allen *et al*, 1990; Sultan *et al*, 1994a). Furthermore, pudendal nerve motor latency following vaginal delivery has been shown to recover in at least two-thirds of women (Snooks *et al*, 1984; Sultan *et al*, 1994a).

Anal endosonography has added a new dimension to understanding the pathogenesis of anal incontinence (Law and Bartram, 1989; Sultan *et al*, 1992). Many patients previously believed to be suffering from pure 'neurogenic' incontinence were subsequently found to have mechanical defects in their sphincter muscle.

Sultan *et al* (1993a) investigated 202 unselected pregnant women prospectively with anal endosonography and anorectal physiology tests during pregnancy and 150 of them 6 weeks postpartum. Antenatally, none of the 79 primiparae who had a vaginal delivery were symptomatic but postnatally 13% had developed defaecatory symptoms (faecal urgency or anal incontinence). Of the 48 multiparae, 23% admitted to defaecatory symptoms which in most women had occurred after the first vaginal delivery. Antenatally, no anal sphincter defects were identified in primiparae but defects were identified in 35% at 6 weeks postpartum (Figures 1 and 2). Defects were identified in 40% of the multiparous women antenatally and only 4% developed a new defect after delivery. This demonstrates that the risk of sphincter damage is greatest during the first vaginal delivery. The 23 women who were delivered by caesarean section remained asymptomatic and no new anal sphincter defects were identified.

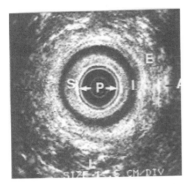

Figure 1. Normal endosono-graphic image (Bruel and Kjaer 7 Mhz rotating endoprobe of the mid anal canal of a nulliparous woman. A=anterior; L=left; E=external anal sphincter; I=internal anal sphincter; P=probe in the anal canal; S=subepithelium

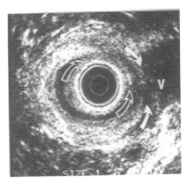

Figure 2. This woman had a forceps delivery and trauma to the anal sphincter was not recognised at delivery. There is a defect in the external (closed arrows) and internal anal sphincter (open arrows). There remains very little muscle anteriorly between the anal canal and the vagina (V)>

Antenatally, 3% of women had a prolonged pudendal nerve terminal motor latency (indicating damage to the fast conducting fibres of the pudendal nerve) but at 6 weeks postpartum this rose to15% (Sultan *et al*, 1994a). However, in contrast to sonographic defects which persisted at 6 months, pudendal nerve latency had recovered in the majority.

On univariate analysis, the presence of an episiotomy, augmentation of labour, epidural analgesia and forceps delivery were associated with the development of anal sphincter defects.

However, on stepwise logistic regression analysis the only independent factor was forceps delivery.

Although only one-third to one-half of the women who had defects were symptomatic, there was a strong correlation between the presence of defects and the development of symptoms. It remains to be established whether women who remained asymptomatic despite the presence of defects are at a higher risk of becoming symptomatic later in life. This may become evident when the long-term follow-up study is completed. To date Donnelly *et al* performed a similar prospective study in Dublin (1995; unpublished data) but using anal vector manometry instead of anal endosonography. They also identified occult anal sphincter defects in 30% of primiparae.

Another area of concern is the poor outcome following primary repair of a third or fourth degree obstetric anal sphincter tear. In four recent studies (Haadem *et al*, 1988; Sorensen *et al*, 1988; Nielsen *et al*, 1992; Sultan *et al*, 1994b) involving a total of 104 women, 29–48% of women reported anal incontinence 3 months to 3 years after primary sphincter repair. Poor outcome was related to the presence of persistent anal sphincter defects rather than pudendal nerve damage (Sultan *et al*, 1994b). Of those women who sustained a third degree tear, 85% were primiparous and 50% were delivered by forceps. Inconsistency in classification of third or fourth degree tears, inappropriate technique of repair and operator inexpertise are major issues that need to be addressed (Sultan *et al*, 1995).

Conclusion

The late presentation by women suffering from longstanding prolapse and incontinence (Norton *et al*, 1987) highlights the embarrassment and misconceptions associated with these physical and socially debilitating conditions. The strong relationship between obstetric trauma and pelvic floor sequelae are now becoming apparent as further technological advances are made in imaging technique. The true magnitude of the problem is only beginning to be appreciated as women are living longer and other aggravating factors, such as ageing, the hormonal effects of the menopause, and progression of pelvic neuropathy, add insult to the initial injury sustained at vaginal delivery. Although a considerable degree of the obstetric trauma sustained is occult, even when injury is recognised and repaired the outcome is not always favourable. Therefore greater effort needs to be directed towards preventing obstetric trauma so as to minimise its sequelae which may not become apparent until late in life. Reduction in the episiotomy rate (Henriksen *et al*, 1994), the use of the vacuum extractor in preference to forceps (Johanson *et al*, 1993; Sultan *et al*, 1993b), caesarean section in selected cases (Sultan and Stanton, 1996) and more focused training for doctors and midwives (Sultan *et al*, 1995) are issues that deserve immediate consideration.

Key points

- Although urinary and faecal incontinence and genital prolapse are the major pelvic floor sequelae of vaginal delivery, their prevalence remains underestimated as women are too embarrassed to seek medical attention.

- The effects of pelvic floor compromise may only manifest late in life even though the major insult usually occurs during the first vaginal delivery.

- The pathogenesis of pelvic floor dysfunction is multifactorial but trauma to the pelvic fascia and connective tissue, pelvic neuropathy and direct muscle injury are the major contributory factors.

- Obstetric factors such as prolonged active second stage of labour, heavy babies, difficult and traumatic delivery and the use of forceps are strongly implicated.

- With continuing research and audit, more focused and intensive training of doctors and midwives and changes in aspects of current obstetric practice we can minimise the devastating social disabilities that can follow vaginal childbirth.

References

Allen RE, Hosker GL, Smith ARB, Warrell DW (1990) Pelvic floor damage and childbirth: a neurophysiological study. *Br J Obstet Gynaecol* **97**: 770–9

Anderson RS (1984) A neurologic element to urinary genuine stress incontinence. *Br J Obstet Gynaecol* **91**: 41–5

Barnick CGW, Cardozo LD (1993) Denervation and reinnervation of the urethral sphincter in the aetiology of genuine stress incontinence: an electromyographic study. *Br J Obstet Gynaecol* **100**: 750–3

Brincat M, Moniz CF, Studd JWW (1993) Sex hormones and skin collagen content in postmenopausal women. *Br Med J* **287**: 1337–8

Deindl FM, Vodusek DB, Hesse U, Schussler B (1994) Pelvic floor activity patterns: comparison of nulliparous continent and parous urinary stress incontinent women. A kinesiological EMG study. *Br J Urol* **73**: 413–17

Gilpin SA, Gosling GA, Smith ARB, Warrell DW (1989) The pathogenesis of genitourinary prolapse and stress incontinence of urine. A histological and histochemical study. *Br J Obstet Gynaecol* **96**: 15–23

Glazener CMA, Abdalla M, Stroud P, Naji S, Templeton A, Russell IT (1995) Postnatal maternal morbidity: extent, causes, prevention and treatment. *Br J Obstet Gynaecol* **102**: 282–7

Haadem K, Ohrlander S, Lingman G (1988) Long-term ailments due to anal sphincter rupture caused by delivery — a hidden problem. *Eur J Obstet Gynecol Reprod Biol* **27**: 27–32

Haadem K, Ling L, Ferno M, Graffner H (1991) Estrogen receptors in the external anal sphincter. *Obstet Gynecol* **164**: 609–10

Henriksen TB, Bek KM, Hedegaard M, Secher NJ (1994) Methods and consequences of change in use of episiotomy. *Br Med J* **309**: 1255–88

Jackson S, Avery N, Eckford S, Shepherd A, Bailey A (1995) Connective tissue analysis in genitourinary prolapse. *Neurourol Urodyn* **14**: 412–14

Johanson RB, Rice C, Doyle M *et al* (1993) A randomised prospective study comparing the new vacuum extractor policy with forceps delivery. *Br J Obstet Gynaecol* **100**: 524–30

Keane DP, Sims TJ, Bailey AJ, Abrams P (1992) Analysis of pelvic floor electromyography and collagen status in premenopausal nulliparous females with genuine stress incontinence. *Neurourol Urodyn* **11**: 308–9

Kirschner-Hermanns R, Wein B, Niehaus S, Schaefer W, Jakse G (1993) The contribution of magnetic resonance imaging of the pelvic floor to the understanding of urinary incontinence. *Br J Urol* **72**: 715–18

Klutke C, Golomb J, Barbaric Z, Raz S (1990) The anatomy of stress incontinence: magnetic resonance imaging of the female bladder neck and urethra. *Urol Neurol Urodyn* **143**: 563–6

Mallett V, Hosker G, Smith ARB, Warrell D (1994) Pelvic floor damage and childbirth: a neurophysiologic follow up study. *Neurourol Urodyn* **13**: 357–8

Laurberg S, Swash M (1989) Effects of ageing on the anorectal sphincters and their innervation. *Dis Colon Rectum* **32**: 737–42

Law PJ, Bartram CI (1989) Anal endosonography: technique and normal anatomy. *Gastrointest Radiol* **14**: 349–53

MacArthur C, Lewis M, Knox EG (1991) *Health After Childbirth.* HMSO, London

McIntosh LJ, Mallett VT, Frahm JM, Richardson DA (1993) Ehlers-Danlos syndrome and gynecologic disorders. *Int Urogynecol J* **4**: 394

Nielsen MB, Hauge C, Rasmussen OO, Pedersen JF, Christiansen J (1992) Anal endosonographic findings in the follow-up of primarily sutured sphincteric ruptures. *Br J Surg* **79**: 104–6

Nichols DH, Randall CL (1983) *Vaginal Surgery.* Williams and Wilkins, Baltimore

Norton P, MacDonald L, Stanton SL (1987) Distress associated with female urinary complaints and delay in seeking treatment. *Neurourol Urodyn* **6**: 170–2

Norton P, Boyd C, Deak S (1992) Collagen synthesis in women with genital prolapse or stress urinary incontinence. *Neurourol Urodyn* **11**: 300–1

Parks AG (1975) Anorectal incontinence. *Proc R Soc Med* **68**: 681–90

Parks AG, Swash M, Urich H (1977) Sphincter denervation in anorectal incontinence and rectal prolapse. *Gut* **18**: 656–65

Shull BL, Benn SJ, Kuehl TJ (1994) Surgical management of prolapse of the anterior vaginal segment: an analysis of support defects, operative morbidity, and anatomic outcome. *Am J Obstet Gynecol* **171**: 1429–39

Sleep J (1991) Perineal care: a series of five randomized controlled trials. In: Robinson S, Thompson AM, eds. *Midwives, Research and Childbirth*. Volume 2. Chapman & Hall, London: 119–251

Smith ARB, Hosker GL,Warrell DW (1989) The role of partial denervation of the pelvic floor in the aetiology of genitourinary prolapse and genuine stress incontinence. A neurophysiological study. *Br J Obstet Gynaecol* **96**: 24–8

Snooks SJ, Swash M, Setchell M, Henry MM (1984) Injury to innervation of pelvic floor sphincter musculature in childbirth. *Lancet* **ii**: 546–50

Snooks SJ, Swash M, Mathers SE, Henry MM (1990) Effect of vaginal delivery on the pelvic floor: a 5-year follow-up. *Br J Surg* **77**: 1358–60

Sorensen SM, Bondesen H, Istre O, Vilmann P (1988) Perineal rupture following vaginal delivery. *Acta Obstet Gynecol Scand* **67**: 315–18

Spence Jones C, Kamm MA, Henry MM, Hudson CN (1994) Bowel dysfunction: a pathogenic factor in uterovaginal prolapse and urinary stress incontinence. *Br J Obstet Gynaecol* **101**: 147–52

Sultan AH, Stanton SL (1996) Preserving the pelvic floor and perineum during childbirth — elective caesarean section? *Br J Obstet Gynaecol* **103** (8): 731–734

Sultan AH, Nicholls RJ, Kamm MA, Hudson CN, Beynon J, Bartram CI (1992) Anal endosonography and correlation with in vitro and in vivo anatomy. *Br J Surg* **80**: 808–11

Sultan AH, Kamm MA, Hudson CN, Thomas JM, Bartram CI (1993a) Anal sphincter disruption during vaginal delivery. *N Engl J Med* **329**:1905–11

Sultan AH, Kamm MA, Bartram CI, Hudson CN (1993b) Anal sphincter trauma during instrumental delivery. A comparison between forceps and vacuum extraction. *Int J Gynecol Obstet* **43**: 263–70

Sultan AH, Kamm MA, Hudson CN (1994a) Pudendal nerve damage during labour: prospective study before and after childbirth. *Br J Obstet Gynaecol* **101**: 22–8

Sultan AH, Kamm MA, Hudson CN, Bartram CI (1994b) Third degree obstetric anal sphincter tears: risk factors and outcome of primary repair. *Br Med J* **308**: 887–91

Sultan AH, Kamm MA, Hudson CN (1995) Obstetric perineal tears: an audit of training. *J Obstet Gynaecol* **15**: 19–23

Thomas TM, Egan M, Walgrove A, Meade TW (1984) The prevalence of faecal and double incontinence. *Comm Med* **6**: 216–20

Ulmsten U, Ekman G, Giertz G, Malmstrom A (1987) Different biochemical composition of connective tissue in continent and stress incontinent women. *Acta Obstet Gynecol Scand* **66**: 455–7

White GR (1912) Cystocele. *JAMA* **853**: 1707–10

Wiskind AK, Creighton SM, Stanton SL (1992) The incidence of genital prolapse after the Burch colposuspension. *Am J Obstet Gynecol* **167(2)**: 399–405

World Health Organisation (1984) *Healthier Mothers and Children Through Family Planning*. Family Planning Programmes. Volume 27. WHO, Geneva: J677